Dr. Frau

Dr. Frau

A Woman Doctor Among the Amish

Grace H. Kaiser

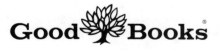

Good Books

Intercourse, PA 17534
800/762-7171
www.goodbks.com

Design by Dawn J. Ranck
Cover illustration by Denny Bond

DR. FRAU
Copyright © 1986, 1997 by Grace H. Kaiser
International Standard Book Number (paperback): 1-56148-216-1
International Standard Book Number (hardcover): 0-934672-34-2
Library of Congress Catalog Card Number: 97-16390
Originally published, 1986
REVISED EDITION, 1997

Library of Congress Cataloging-in-Publication Data

Kaiser, Grace H.
    Dr. Frau : a woman doctor among the Amish / Grace H.
Kaiser. -- Rev. ed.
        p. cm.
    ISBN: 1-56148-216-1
    1. Obstetricians--Pennsylvania--Lancaster County--
Biography. 2. Osteopathic physicians--Pennsylvania--
Lancaster County--Biography. 3. Gynecologists--
Pennsylvania--Lancaster County--Biography. 4. Amish--
Pennsylvania--Lancaster County--Social life and customs.
I. Title.
RG76.K34A33 1997
610'.92--dc21
[B]   97-16390
                                                      CIP

Author's Note

The intent of DR. FRAU is entertainment. Insight into the Amish and Mennonite cultures is an intended bonus.

If readers believe they recognize characters, perhaps themselves, they are right. But look again. Places and situations are as mixed as tickets in a raffle barrel. All names are fictitious. If there is, or ever was, a covered bridge at Harristown, I never saw or heard of it. If anyone feels omitted, search. A part of you, or our relationship, is included. No person or group is preferred above another. I enjoyed them all.

Time makes little change in the Plain People. Their lifestyles, manners, beliefs persist as they have for generations. The people live in a yesterday culture that coexists with tomorrow's world.

Acknowledgments

To Dorothy Lykes for her inspiration
and guidance from the day
I attended her first class;
To Marguerite Noble, author, grammarian,
for her unlimited assistance;
To the Monday Critique Group
for listening, patience, and help.

Table of Contents

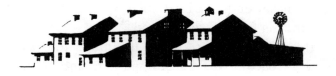

1.
Surrogate Mother

Melvin King limped across the kitchen with the air of a man in control of his world. He paused in the kettlehouse doorway. The rust-pocked Coleman lantern swinging from his twisted left arm bleated a hole into the black predawn.

"I'll be in the barn doin' the milkin'. If you need me, set the lamp in the window," he said, chomping a burned-out matchstick. He looked toward the slow-sizzling slabs of mush frying in a pan on the gas stove. "Can you watch that mush? Turn it when it gets brown."

I nodded and wished he would leave. The night had been long and rough. My thoughts were on the worn couch at the other end of the kitchen.

Melvin stopped. "Oh yes, if the kids come down, send them over to Mom's." He pointed to the outline of a small frame house barely visible across the barnyard.

He hobbled off before the impact of his words registered in my weary head. I had often been called out of bed to sit with a laboring wife, but this was the first time I had been assigned household chores. I sat at the table surveying my new domain.

The night had been short on sleep and long on work when Melvin had telephoned. Having fallen into bed at 1:30 a.m. after attending a birth near Mascot, I had been in no mood for his fun or jovial mood.

"Yes, this is Dr. Kaiser," I had mumbled into the telephone, eyes closed. I was determined to maintain that state of semiconsciousness allowing my return to sleep.

"That you, Grace?" the snappy voice repeated.

"Yes."

"Know who this is?"

"No, and I don't play guessing games. It's the middle of the night. Who are you?"

"We'll be needin' you soon," returned the too cheerful answer.

"Yes, who will?" I shivered and squirmed deeper into the down comforter, carrying the telephone with me.

"Rebecca will. This is Melvin King below Intercourse, toward Harristown, second farm across the covered bridge."

Melvin King was a farmer who conducted his family and acres with firm purpose. Like all Amish, unless tenanting farms not owned by their people, he had no telephone.

The telephone held such fascination for Melvin that it was conducive to entertainment. I was in no mood for it. He had probably gone to bed at 8:30 the night before.

I risked opening one eye to look at the ceiling. The alarm clock projected 3:30 a.m. through a hole in its plastic top. I would put Melvin off several hours.

"This is just a warning then," I said. "Call me back after you finish milking and let me know how she feels." I began to hang up.

"Rebecca thought you oughta come soon. Her pains are every 15 minutes and getting harder. Better not wait 'til morning."

"I'll be out soon." Submissively, I fumbled the phone onto its cradle. The clock glared 3:37. Almost milking time. Melvin probably wants me to speed up Rebecca's labor, or tell him it is okay for him to go to the barn. Every Amish kitchen has a couch. I could nap on it.

Afraid of falling asleep, I dragged myself from beneath warm covers and groped for the pile of clothes on the rocking chair beside the bed.

"I'm going out again. Call me on the car phone and beeper," I half shouted to my husband, attempting to reach his conscious level.

"You coming in or going out?" the mound under the covers muttered.

"Been in, going out again," I repeated, raising my voice several decibels.

"Okay, good luck." The lump shifted, hunting a quieter place.

I never knew how much he heard, but he always located me if necessary.

In the car the chill of late winter air and the challenge of potholes awakened me. I hoped Rebecca would be ready for her home birthing when I arrived.

Early morning prior to milking time was a period of what I called "barn panic." A herdsman, torn between obligation to his laboring wife in the house and milk-laden cows in the barn, faced a true dilemma. This was worsened by a milk truck which usually arrived on schedule. Sometimes I suspected that I filled the role of a convenient wife-sitter.

It was still black night when I swung around the last pot-
hole and onto Kings' gravel lane. A white board fence ran
beside the drive, ending in the yard near the old brick
farmhouse. I parked under a giant maple, grotesque in winter nudity. Its whitewashed trunk stood out boldly in the
headlights.

March frost crackled beneath my boots like eggshells on
the concrete walk. I shone my flashlight on the icy slabs,
tilted by sprawling roots of the old tree.

Melvin stood stocking-footed in the kettlehouse doorway, waving a Coleman lantern into the night. He shifted
a gnawed toothpick from one side of his mouth to the
other. "I wonder if you better park there. The milk truck
will be comin' in after 'while."

"How soon?" I was well up the long walk.

"Seven to seven-thirty."

"Hope I won't be here that long. Good morning,
Melvin."

I wiped my boots on the burlap-bag footmat and followed the swaying lantern through the kettlehouse. We
passed shadowed outlines of pies, puddings, and pans of
congealed cornmeal mush sitting on the wooden lid of the
great bricked-in iron kettle used to heat Monday's wash
water or cook meat at butchering time.

Melvin cast a sparse shadow. He walked with a lurch
and carried his lantern at a peculiar angle. Five years ago
he had slipped from a load of hay and landed beneath the
iron wagon wheels. I remember him lying between the
windrows of dried alfalfa while awaiting the Paradise
Community Ambulance. His left arm had been twisted and
bleeding; bones pierced the skin of his lower leg. While
administering first aid I had wondered if the limb could be

saved. Concerned about hospital costs and his farm, he remained in the Lancaster hospital only until he was certain Rebecca could care for him. Then he signed his own discharge and went home. Deformities did not slow his steps.

I followed Melvin's rocking form through the large kitchen and into the adjoining bedroom where Rebecca lay beneath a pile of quilts.

"Hello, doctor. Guess I'm in no hurry." Rebecca's globular face smiled creases and dimples, put there by many helpings of potatoes and gravy. A long thin scar extended from her right ear to her chin. At age nine she had been thrown from her father's spring wagon when a young horse bolted and ran away.

Her dentures did not fit well, clipping her words short. I could only imagine the result of a strong sneeze. If she had ever been pretty it was not important. When not ill she worked hard, mothering Melvin's and her five children. Rebecca was always pleasant, despite constant attention to her many physical complaints. If she was careless with housework or "felt poorly" at times, it was overlooked by her family.

Rebecca lay as limp as yesterday's lettuce leaf in an old oak bed with high headboard and sagging mattress. It was cold in the room. The fires had been banked for the night. My patient's white muslin nightcap, tied beneath a generous chin, enclosed her pale face on the white bolster. When I peeled back the log cabin quilt to examine her, pink sheet blankets lined the bed.

"How soon do you think?" Melvin asked. He anxiously chewed his toothpick and fidgeted with his black socks which had fallen from under the legs of his grey-black

broadfalls. The home-sewn pants of Amish men and boys
have buttons across the top. Suspenders, worn over plain
colored shirts of green, blue, pink, brown, or lavender, support the wide-waisted pants. Sunday pants are black and
the shirts white.

"The delivery won't be for awhile. I'll go home again," I
answered, repacking my bag. "How far does Melvin have
to go to the telephone?"

"He has to walk to the pay phone at Osceola Mill, about
three-fourths of a mile," Rebecca answered, grimacing with
a contraction.

I laid a hand gently on her mounded abdomen, palpat-
ing only a mild hardening of its surface. Not much of a contraction, I thought.

"I'll have to go to the barn soon," Melvin said, jostling
his soggy toothpick. "Remember how fast she went with
her second baby? You hardly made it through that door."

His beard shone bright orange in the glow of lamplight.
Pushing a clump of amber hair from his narrow face, he
pleaded. "It's better she's not alone. You can rest on the
kitchen couch."

"Okay, Melvin, but make it warmer in here," I said,
accepting a blanket and heading for the kitchen. His argu-
ment was justified, for several times I had left a patient in
what I believed to be early labor and returned to find a
panicked husband and an excited mother with a baby in
her bed.

I know of no Amish kitchen without its infamous couch,
often in a state of decline and decay. They appear to be the
most popular piece of furniture. The housewife usually
recovers them in shades of plain blue, gray, or maroon.
House dogs, as well as ensnared doctors, sleep on the

chunky cushions. On these couches with their lumps and bumps, the children play, spill milk from their bottles, and wet their pants. The King couch was typical. It also had a strong barn odor due to a row of work shoes sitting under its end near the stove.

I always brought coats long enough to use for a cover when there were no blankets. Many nights I rolled my coat up for a pillow. Sometimes I tossed restlessly in bed at home, but I could sleep instantly when called out to one of these remarkable pallets.

Melvin obligingly turned up the propane heater in the bedroom, conversing with his wife in Pennsylvania Dutch, the mother tongue of the Amish, a German dialect, mingled with English words. Then he shook down the fire in the kitchen stove, jabbed it vigorously with a long poker and poured on coal from a scuttle before opening the draft. The new coal crackled and sent whiffs of sulphur into the room before he closed the iron door.

"Guess I'll go to the barn and do the feedin'," Melvin said, glancing at a gilt-trimmed mantel clock. He sat in his captain's chair at the head of the table, moving a barn-burner between his lips as he pulled a pair of dirt-caked shoes from under the couch.

He picked a faded gray jacket and worn broad-brimmed black hat from hooks behind the stove. "I'll be back in 45 minutes to check on things." Removing the match from pinched lips, he lit a barn lantern.

I raised a green window shade and watched Melvin disappear into the black cavernous cow stable.

After several turns on the couch, I mapped its lumps and springs. It seemed I had barely settled between them when Melvin stomped back into the kitchen.

"Feedin's done. Anything happenin' here?" he asked in high spirits, pinching a stalk of timothy hay between his teeth.

"I think things will change soon," Rebecca called from her bed. "Don't let the doctor go home."

"Might as well start the milking then." He took the draft off the stove.

"How many cows do you milk?" I asked, examining Rebecca. She had changed very little. Perhaps her contractions were stronger. At the present rate I calculated several hours before birthing.

"Twenty-seven just now. It takes 'bout an hour and a half by myself." He munched his hay stem and laughed boyishly. "Goes faster when Becky helps—but it looks like she's started her vacation." The thought of his wife's vacation lit his face with a blush.

Instead of returning to the barn, Melvin meticulously scrubbed his hands in the kitchen wash sink beside the kettlehouse door and wiped them on a towel hanging over a nail in the corner. An embroidered huck towel with blue crocheted edging hung over a dowel beneath a mirrored medicine cabinet, but it was for decoration only.

Melvin picked a match from a glass dish on the gas stove and lit a burner beneath an iron skillet from the pantry. I watched his coarse hands deftly cut thick slices of cornmeal mush from a pan and lay them onto the hot lard which sputtered and bounced as each piece touched the fat. He turned the gas low, substituted the burned match for his timothy, and was off to the barn before I could respond to my household instructions.

I sat at the long kitchen table covered with flowered oilcloth. Was this why I had spent those years in medical school? I was both annoyed and amused. Suppose Melvin, after church or at family gatherings, should pass this incident through the *freundschaft?* If better judgment had prevailed, I would have gone home to bed.

Amish homes never ceased to interest me. Behind the coal stove a row of black coats hung on metal hooks. Eight calendars of five years' variation hung along the walls. One showed the current month. Rebecca rehung them after spring and fall housecleaning because she liked the colorful pictures: snow-covered mountains, kittens in a yarn basket, puppies in a box, farm scenes across the nation. I smiled, recalling the many notes, pencil-scrawled on the backs of expired calendar pages, I had received from rural mailboxes.

On the wall above the table, a homemade letter holder held a recent issue of the religious publication, *Family Life;* a copy of *The Sugar Creek Budget,* an Amish newspaper; and several local papers.

By the shadowed light of the lantern hanging from the ceiling hook above the table, I noticed that the stone-patterned linoleum was worn bare-brown before the sink and gas stove. A flat brass strip ribboned the flooring at its seam.

Where I had raised the shades at the north windows, I could see the outline of my car silhouetted against the glow from the stable casements. I heard the steady pant of the diesel engine and knew Melvin was busy milking.

Rebecca shuffled through the kitchen en route to the bathroom beside the kettlehouse. She slid her feet as if this, perhaps her last trip out of bed for some time, was a supreme effort.

I considered my mix of roles with humor and tried to decide whether to admire Melvin for either his naiveté or his cunning. Had I been ambushed or had events fallen into place by guided convenience?

My musings were interrupted by scuffling feet in a closed stairway. The door opened and seven-year-old Johnny stepped wide-eyed into the room. He stopped on the bottom step, blinking big brown eyes on seeing a non-Amish stranger in the kitchen. Dressed in gray broadfalls and green shirt, he was a miniature Melvin in copper curls.

"Geh zu Dat im barn, Johnny," Rebecca called from her bed.

Without a questioning word or glance he picked out a pair of black shoes and stockings from the assortment and sat on the couch to put them on. He looked at his mother in mute astonishment, buttoned on a jacket, grabbed a broadbrim and ran to the barn.

"Another one," I called as Aaron, age five, stepped into the room. He stared, rubbing his eyes with chubby fists, then sidled along the wall to the line of shoes. Light brown hair, cut Dutchboy style like his father's and brother's, framed a child face that seriously considered me from every angle. I wondered how he pulled on socks and tied his shoes, for he stared at me constantly.

Rebecca chatted to him in Dutch, the only tongue he knew. He slid slowly along the wall to the bedroom, bewildered at seeing his mother there instead of in the barn or getting breakfast. With unquestioning obedience, he, too, dressed and ran to the barn.

"I tell them I'm sick today, and the 'Dr. Frau' is here to make me better," Rebecca said.

"Guten Morgen," I greeted a little girl in a long muslin nightdress when she opened the stair door. She slid quietly around me and darted into the bedroom. Long red

braids bounced over the nightcap hanging along her neck by its string.

"Susie is four. She can dress herself," Rebecca called. "Will you tie her shoes? We'll send her over to Mom's as soon as Mary gets up."

Thoughts of the couch and a nap vanished. My patient lay on her pillows while I tied Susie's shoes and buttoned the back of her dress. Uncomprehending, she watched everything, allowing me to help her. If I had knotted her shoes together or buttoned her dress crooked I wondered if she would have objected. She did not speak a word. Her rewarding smile transcended language.

A scratching, fumbling sound came from the stairwell as I hung Susie's nightgown on a hook. Behind the door stood a chubby child in pajamas and nightcap. A foreigner at such close range filled her black eyes with fright. She allowed me to pick her up.

Rebecca would not move from her bed. I tossed Mary's malodorous diaper into the washbowl with a splat and dressed the two-year-old with clothes like Susie's—a green dress, black ankle-high shoes, and black stockings held below the knees with bands of white elastic. I helped the girls into black jackets and lavender bonnets. They held hands, walking toward their grandmother's house where a lamp shone in her kitchen window.

The mush! Black smoke filled the kitchen. I ran to the stove. A few pieces were burned. I turned the slices and hurried back to Rebecca, who began to groan with each contraction. On examination, I saw she was still far from delivery.

A cushioned rocking chair near the stove looked good. I sank into it with a quiet groan.

"Do I hear a baby crying?" I asked, lifting my head to hear more clearly.

"Rachel must be awake. We put her upstairs with the other children last night for the first time. You'll find her in the room over the kitchen." Rebecca lifted her head to be sure I understood.

I groped my way up the dim stairway to the warmest bedroom, shared by the little girls. The baby stomped around a soggy crib complaining in a deafening voice. When she saw me, her protest increased. She was wet and reeked of the brown which stained her diaper. Balancing her on one arm, I carried the squalling baby downstairs, threw the messed diaper on top of Mary's and hunted a washcloth.

The miserable moppet screamed and struggled as I rediapered and dressed her. Tears of fright rolled over her fat cheeks. She yelled louder when I tried to wipe her nose. Beneath her nightcap, wisps of red baby hair escaped the soft lead bobbies used to roll the loose strands from her face. Peace finally came when I gave her two crackers and set her in a far corner.

Most women, birthing at home, go about their housework as long as possible. But Rebecca had begun her vacation at the first labor twinge. She seemed to believe that caring for more than herself and the new baby, at least for several weeks, would be unthinkable.

It was nearly full daylight when furious shouting came from the driveway. I reached the window in time to see a long stainless steel milk truck back slowly up the driveway. Melvin ran beside the truck shouting and waving his arms. Too late. A crunch of steel on steel. The rear of my station wagon lifted, folded. Dust flew. The driver felt the impact, pulled forward, and jumped out of the cab. He and Melvin inspected the damages. I ran out, too.

"We'll get it fixed. Couldn't see it there. We'll fix it," the driver said, excited.

We talked about insurance and repairs. The milkman loaded his truck from the bulk tank. Melvin and I went to the house.

Melvin allowed nothing to interfere with the satisfaction of his appetite. I declined breakfast. He fried slices of puddins (fatty pork fried crisp and drained). Fascinated, I watched him put the cracklings, fried mush, and two poached eggs in a soup plate of stewed crackers (saltines soaked in hot milk). Getting breakfast seemed routine to him.

Baby Rachel clung to her father's legs until he set her in a wooden high chair beside him. Before they ate, Melvin folded the baby's hands in her lap, and they both bowed their heads silently before eating. He shared his breakfast by feeding Rachel from his spoon or laying bits of shoo-fly pie on her tray. Melvin dunked each spoonful of his pie in coffee.

They repeated the silent prayer when they finished eating. Melvin added his dishes to a stack that had accumulated in the sink.

It was time to attend the patient. For the past hour she had moved from her mattress only to use a white enamel chamber bucket which she dragged from under the bed with a clatter.

Melvin and I talked, cajoled, and worked, coaxing Rebecca through a slow labor. He was his usual cheerful self, expecting, not demanding. He encouraged his wife without raising his voice, insisting she cooperate. We delivered a nine-pound baby boy.

When I packed my bag at 10 o'clock, Melvin tore a page from one of the old calendars. "I'll write a note to brother John's. You'll be passin' their place. They'll send their daughter Mary Ann over as hired girl 'til I fetch Annie Petersheim for nurse. Drive in and blow your horn. They'll run out." He folded the note into a square.

I walked past the griddle of cold fried mush, past the washbowl of dirty diapers and the sinkful of waiting dishes, through the kettlehouse to my crinkled car.

Again Melvin stood stocking-footed in the doorway. Removing the toothpick from between his lips, he leaned over the concrete walk. "See you next time," he called.

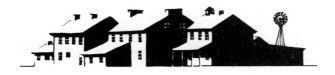

2.
Ezra's Baby

Babies, blunders, and Ezra King were far from my mind as I nested a 20-pound turkey, stuffed with oyster dressing, in the oven. The automatic timer read 3:00 a.m. I set stewed cranberries, cooked giblets, and fresh pumpkin pie in the refrigerator. Working furiously since the end of evening office hours, I knew my Thanksgiving dinner would be as tasty as any housewife's.

The last sticky pan hit the sink at half-past collapse time—11:30 p.m. Bing Jake's Ezra phoned. Mattie would be ready to birth her baby in about an hour.

Nancy Pritchard, student nurse and our former babysitter, had asked to go along on a home birth. Within minutes she dressed and walked across two backyards.

I opened the oven for a final admiring peek. Patting the soft turkey breast, I imagined the aroma of onions and sage filtering into our upstairs bedroom by morning.

Identity and genealogy, important to the Amish, are not easy to follow. With so much repetition of names and initials, nicknames are common.

Ezra's father, Jake King, was a white-bearded patriarch when I moved to New Holland. He fathered 16 children, had innumerable grandchildren, and as many great-grand-children. During Jake and Lydia's family years, the Lancaster *Intelligencer Journal* made a typographical error in the birth column. "King" was misprinted "Bing." Thereafter he was "Bing Jake." His children were Bing Jake's Mary, Bing Jake's Jake, etc. Grandchildren became Bing Jake's Jake's Mary . . ., Barbara, . . . Jake, and so on.

Bing Jake's Ezra met Nancy and me at their sun porch door. Standing three steps above us in the glare of a Coleman lantern, Ezra wore a black bushy beard that appeared too heavy for his narrow face. He seemed taller and thinner than when he visited the office with Mattie.

"What you doin' here, Grace?" Ezra's Adam's apple bob-bled above a pink shirt collar. "Who called you?"

"You didn't call me?" I was sure the man had said Ezra King at Centerville. Confused dismay must have shown as I turned to leave.

"Well, as long as you're here you can stay and deliver Mattie." He could not hide a wide grin as he hung the lantern above the kitchen table. It swayed several minutes, dancing our silhouettes along the blue wall.

I was angry with Ezra and embarrassed at having fallen prey to one of his capers. Teasing seemed his greatest delight. The first time he brought Mattie into my office he had been quiet and glum.

"What's the trouble?" I asked, knowing him as talkative and happy.

"Mattie had an accident." His heavy brows furrowed behind wispy bangs and nearly hid the brown eyes usually shining with mischief.

"What happened?" I leaned forward to inspect Mattie. She was expressionless, but appeared healthy and uninjured.

"She got pregnant," Ezra blurted. He snorted and guffawed, enjoying my concern.

It was typical of Bing Jake's boys' humor. They were pranksters. Several times I heard the story of a young couple who parked their Volkswagen along a farm lane near Centerville. The lovers walked into the cornfield. When they returned, the rear axle had been lifted onto field stones. The only people in sight were iron-faced men rocking on the King porch.

When Nancy and I settled into cushioned rockers, I resolved to be wary of my jokester host. He was an honest, astute farmer, successful in dairy and field, but I did not trust his humor.

"Don't think I'll keep you long," Mattie said, stopping to rub her abdomen. She smiled, showing a set of dentures with gums brighter pink than I had ever seen.

I was sure she laid a generous table and enjoyed everything she cooked. By appearance, it was difficult to tell she was pregnant until she neared term. At 36, her scalp was nearly bare around her face from years of twisting her hair into a tight knot behind her head. The hair roots had been destroyed. But the hair that was left mingled gray and brown along the edge of her cap.

Mattie was always quiet and soft-spoken, probably her defense against Ezra's talkative habits. She was an old friend. I had delivered five of her seven children and had seen them through colds, flu, and childhood diseases. The King children, as in most Amish families, did not receive "baby shots."

Mattie scuffed around her tidy kitchen in brown felt slippers. She stopped to time contractions or pick a paper scrap from the linoleum. Gold-framed glasses gave her round face a dignity worthy of her matriarchal domain.

I followed her with envy, remembering my kitchen clutter. Mattie's counter tops were bare of the canister set, blender, toaster, mixer, and can opener that littered mine. Where had I gone awry with order and efficiency?

The car's horn broke my musings. I ran through the porch and across the yard before the telephone operator could blow it again. It was Pete calling. Another patient, Marvin Burkholder's wife, near Reamstown, needed me as soon as possible.

"Please call them back and say I'll be there in about an hour," I said, crossing my fingers. "I wish patients would give more warning and not expect me always to be home," I muttered to my husband. It seemed they all hated to crawl out of warm beds to find a telephone, despite my instructions.

It was difficult to resume small talk with Ezra and Mattie. She leisurely paced the kitchen. Her generous home-sewn housecoat, swaying around thick ankles, amplified her shapelessness.

Repeatedly I looked at the battery-powered clock behind the table. Fifteen minutes. Katherine needed me, but I could not leave Mattie. False alarms were common. Perhaps Katherine only imagined she needed me. On the other hand, most women after several births were dependable estimators. Hurry, Mattie, I secretly urged.

Ten minutes later Mattie went to bed. I gloved and waited. The car horn blew two long reverberating blasts into the night and the quiet crossroad homes. The noise would probably awaken residents snuggled in beds. They might stir, smile, nudge a spouse, knowing that Mattie and Ezra "had the doctor." Ezra would receive the teasing.

There was no time to answer the telephone. Within moments, a fat baby lay on the bed. It cried and flexed arms and legs tightly against its body. Quickly, I cut the cord and handed the baby to Nancy, head first. Two large soft bulges protruded between its thighs.

"It's a boy," I said.

Between delivery of baby and placenta, two more echoing beeps shook Centerville. I dashed to the telephone.

"Marvin says it's urgent," Pete reported. "Oh, yes, Harvey Martin's wife is in labor, too. They'll call again."

I raced back to Mattie, expressed the placenta, and gave postpartum instructions while Nancy dressed the baby and put it in a small crib. Ezra received my apologies for leaving the cleanup to him.

There is no direct route between Centerville and Reamstown. I straightened many curves. Nancy buckled her seat belt and hung on.

We left the Amish farm area and entered predominately Old Order Mennonite country. In these parts, farmers often use iron-wheeled tractors as well as horses. Many houses have telephones; some have no running water. Homes range from primitive to finely papered and electrified.

Marvin heard us coming. He peered into the night, filling the kitchen doorway in faded Levis.

"Hurry, hurry, she's havin' it," he called.

Flashlight in one hand, bag in the other, Nancy at my heels, I ran through the yard and into the bedroom beyond the kitchen.

"Come on, it's comin'," Katherine shouted. She panted furiously.

A head of black hear bulged the perineum. With only time to glove I guided a baby girl onto the mattress.

"Just in time," I gasped, not recovered from my sprint.

Nancy opened a sterile pack, and I finished my work while she cleaned and dressed the baby.

Katherine smiled, relieved that we had arrived before the birth. Age 40, she had never delivered any of her 11 children without a doctor.

"Thought I was gonna get the job tonight," Marvin laughed. He slid into a chair. "I'm sure relieved you got here."

The patient smiled a toothless grin, slapped a hand to her mouth and reached into a cup on the bedside table.

"It all worked out okay," she said with a lisp.

Katherine's placenta slithered into the plastic basin as the car telephone came to life again.

"Harvey S. Martin wants you soon as possible. Alta called this time."

Alta was expecting her second baby, and I wanted to be present at her first home birth. We had only four miles instead of the 15 of this last trip.

I gave Katherine quick instructions and left cleanup to Marvin.

"Where's the next baby stop?" he asked.

"Would you have wanted me to tell on *you*?"

"Well, no." He grinned, shaking a burly head.

"Better hurry. I know what it's like to hold back," Katherine said.

Katherine and Marvin would be alone until morning. A telephone on the kitchen wall, beside the lead-lined dry sink with a water bucket and dipper, provided a lifeline to the world.

"If you have any problems or questions, call immediately," I warned, worried about leaving a patient so soon after birthing. Mattie and Katherine were both veterans. They knew the rules: check and rub the pineapple above the pubis every five minutes for an hour, nurse the baby if it cries, call the doctor if in doubt.

When we saw Alta waiting under the porch light we knew her delivery was not imminent. She took us through a wainscoted kitchen. Roller-painted pink flowers on amber plaster brightened the wall above the dark wood.

I watched Alta, slim and lithe except for her pregnant bulge, and wondered how she would look at 38. Would she be a sack with a string around her middle? Would her face be as heavy and creased as those of the last two patients? How many children would she birth? Would the roses on the newly papered bedroom wall still be there, faded and peeling?

Nancy and I sat with Alta several hours. She was glad to hear about Katherine and Marvin, members of the same church. Labor's flush accented her flashing blue eyes. She was young and pretty.

At four o'clock we awoke Harvey upstairs. He rubbed his eyes and staggered across the room. "I have to plow today. Can't stay up all night and walk behind the horses all day," he said.

Harvey was typical of many young Mennonite boys seen riding bicycles around the countryside any Sunday afternoon. His carousing ended when he married Alta, but his bike would provide transportation most of his life.

With thick fingers he pushed a hunk of black hair away from his bright eyes. I understood why he had won Alta's heart. He was pleasant, tall and handsome, clean-shaven, and neat. He filled only half a doorway. White elastic suspenders held his black Sunday pants over the white shirt.

Harvey had little to say, sitting beside Alta during her first home delivery. Had we spoken Pennsylvania Dutch I imagine he would have been more at ease. He laid a hand gently on his wife's shoulder and stroked her arm.

The Martins were pleased with a son. I sutured a small episiotomy, made Alta comfortable, and discussed postpartum care while Nancy dressed the baby.

During our ride home, Nancy and I reviewed the night's work: three uneventful deliveries with healthy babies. We had attended them all. Three families had reason to be thankful on the holiday.

Best of all, Ezra had not gotten the best of us.

I walked through my kitchen at 6:00 a.m. and tiptoed into our bedroom, inhaling onions and sage.

"You just getting in?" Pete rose from the pile of covers. "Ezra called an hour or so after you left there."

"I was afraid I left Mattie too soon."

"No, it's the baby. After you left, it cried. When Ezra picked it up to change the diaper he got a shock."

"For goodness sake. Is the baby okay?"

"He carried the baby to Mattie, 'Look, this baby's a girl.' Ezra went to the phone so you'd know not to report it wrong."

Nancy knew she had dressed a girl but said nothing. She thought I wanted to repay a score with Ezra.

I would hear about this forever. Had it been Marvin or Harvey, they would have flashed a smile and then forgotten. Not Ezra. From then on, our conversations never omitted the questions of determining a girl baby from a boy.

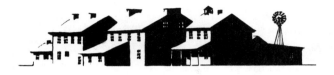

3.
Cherry Picking

The day I took Suvilla Riehl to the cherry orchard, thoughts about my professional reputation were as remote as icebergs from the equator.

In Lancaster County the month of June slides in on the heels of May with little more notice than the rip of a calendar page and an increased pace of daily chores. House, garden, and fields are busy from first light until the last sun ray sets on hay rake and hoe.

June is both beginning and ending, a month of planting and harvest. Warm balmy days and cold nights dissolve into the sultry days and restless nights of torrid July.

Tractors churn and pant in many fields. Among Amish and many Mennonite farmers, great hairy horses or plucky mules, their heads bobbing before heavy loads, traverse patchwork hills and valleys. Defying thunderheads gathering on the horizon, teams plod belly-deep in green. They move to the rhythm of whirring mowers, lopping grasses that fall to sweet hay. Late corn patches await planting.

Young tobacco plants compete for space with weeds, needing hoe and cultivator. Men hitch four or six animals to binders, replacing modern rubber-tired wheels with older iron ones, and cut undulating yellow grain into sheaves.

The clean straight-rowed gardens of farm women are works of art. After-supper weeding and hoeing is rewarded with abundant yields of strawberries, raspberries, and peas. There is plenty for the families' frozen food lockers at Kauffman's or Tri-Town Market. Housewives fill canning jars and set extra berries on roadside tables with bunches of beets, new potatoes, spring onions, and rhubarb. These road stands put money in apron pockets and delight gardenless town people.

Immaculate produce patches are at their best in June. Kitchens are as busy as the fields. Prodigious tables feed hungry field hands. Women, who don't drive slaving horses, toil in the kitchen to meet the calendar of harvest.

Toward the last of June, lustrous cherries hang thick and sweet on trees. Orchard men fix days for public picking. Buckets, tubs, and lard cans are readied for the event. Plans are laid and alarm clocks set for early rising.

I enjoyed planning, picking, and preparing a long row of canned cherries on our cellar shelves. By June the last year's jars were empty, and I hungered for the fresh ripe fruit. The night before picking I put plastic buckets in the car, set the alarm for 4:45 a.m. and hoped no doctor call altered my ambitions.

It was still dark when the ringing began. I punched the alarm. The ringing continued. "4:00 a.m." focused on the ceiling from the clock when I opened one eye. I fumbled the phone into bed.

"This is Isaiah Riehl. Better come see Suvilla."

"Now? How soon?"

"No hurry, but she means business."

"Okay. I'll be over." No cherries today, I thought. Oh, well, another picking next week. I'll try again.

I telephoned Anna, my office nurse. She was disgustingly awake when I pulled to her curb. "Good morning," I mumbled. "Isaiah Riehl this time."

"Not far; only Old Philly Pike near Intercourse," she said, climbing into the station wagon.

Along the Riehl lane our headlights shone on rows of young corn, cabbages, and string beans. A cottontail scampered between carrots and peas. Heavy dew shrouded everything.

Suvilla, barefooted, greeted us at the kettlehouse door. With a kerosene lamp she guided us up the uneven concrete walk and under a lumpy trunked maple. A massive blue nightgown swept her ankles, puffed heavily from the pressure of late pregnancy. Below the nightie's wide hem, tortuous veins stood out like swollen rivers. The seersucker gown ballooned Suvilla's generous figure as we followed her into the kitchen.

"A nice summer day. I'm too busy now to have a baby," she laughed blithely. Her rotund face was framed by a muslin nightcap tied under one chin.

"We're ready to deliver this baby," I said, following her fluttering lamp into the bedroom.

"Yes, let's get this party over before it gets hot." Suvilla lay on her bed prepared with plastic and a homemade newspaper pad. "Looks like I'll have vacation during busy season this year."

I turned to Anna after examining Suvilla. "She's far from

ready. We'll watch her for an hour. If she doesn't make any progress, we'll leave."

"I'm sure it'll come today," Suvilla said, nodding toward a farm I knew lay behind the hill. "We sent the kids over to Brother Jake's before you came." Her broad face layered into creased smiles.

Suvilla waddled into the parlor and dragged two cushioned rocking chairs into the kitchen. Each loose cushion was artfully needlepointed in red, blue, and green flowers on a black background. We settled into their comfort for an hour's wait.

Our patient flowed around her kitchen, busy with small chores. She swept the brick-patterned Congoleum, worn bare before the sink and doorways. By the dim light she seemed shapeless, picking up toys from a corner and putting dishes from the drainboard into the cupboard. Suvilla had a witty tongue and a merry twinkle in her brown eyes. Each time she said anything amusing her pug nose wrinkled. Her laughter was so contagious that we chuckled helplessly at her.

The first time I met Suvilla, she worked as a hired girl for her brother Ben on a farm between Monterey and Mascot. She nursed for Ben's wife Sara after the birth of a baby.

"Don't look for any business from me," she had said. "I'll stay single and happy, thank you. No babies for me."

Suvilla giggled when I recalled her words.

"I got a good man and seven healthy kids. I'm not sorry," she said, grins wrinkling her bright eyes to a squint.

She had sat with other single women in their section of Amish church when Isaiah A. Riehl, a bachelor harnessmaker from the village of Intercourse, asked her to marry him.

"Now I'm about to take a vacation, with three bushels of peas to pick and hull, 50 feet of strawberries ready, and string beans by the basket. The twins are 10; the next one's nearly nine. They're good help, and, of course, Mom will come over."

Headlights moved out from a side road across the street.

"There go one of the Kauffmans to the orchard," I said, walking to a front window.

"Yes, I planned to pick cherries today," Suvilla said with resignation. "Maybe Isaiah will pick next week for us."

"I wanted to pick today, too," I said. "My buckets are in the car. Suvilla, you're still in very early labor. Do you feel like going? We could all go."

"Could I? It's only half-a-mile. I couldn't have the doctor any closer," she chuckled. "What would people say?"

"Other people need not know. There will be plenty of cherries close to the ground if we go now. We'll stick close together and I'll help you. It will be hours before you deliver."

"You've scared my labor away. Let's go." Suvilla laughed heartily at the thought of fooling friends by picking cherries while in labor. A multitude of people would pick that morning. The prospect of telling about it later and watching shocked expressions delighted her most.

Suvilla quickly padded into the bedroom and reappeared so fast I wondered what she had, or had not, put on under the pink dress she closed down the front with straight pins. Her muslin nightcap had been replaced by a white organdy covering tied in a neat bow beneath her chins and pinned on top to a black cotton ribbon circumscribing her head. She carried shoes and black stockings in

one hand and picked up a nest of buckets from the kettlehouse with the other.

"I'll put these on in the car," she said, still chuckling.
More straight pins fastened a pink apron.

"Behave yourself," I warned. "Let us know any time you
want to come home."

Suvilla rushed out to a small barn to tell Isaiah of our
plans. When she returned she was not smiling. "He does-
n't think much of the idea. Says he might as well have gone
to work today. We'll see."

Although Suvilla was in early light labor, my concern
was for more than her health. I sensed that I was about to
destroy the sanctity, mystery, and privacy of labor and
birth. This culture was gravely discreet. working at home
until ready to lie down and give birth was acceptable, but
to go out into a public place . . .

In Amish one-room schools, sex education is not taught.
Children are not told when a woman becomes pregnant or
goes into labor. As birthing time nears, children are sent to
a neighbor, to the barn, or to the other end of the house
where grandparents, Mommy and Dawdy, usually live.
Only when God's new gift lies beside its mother are children permitted to share the family joy.

Suvilla was too modest to tell anyone in the orchard
about her labor. But what of tomorrow and next week? She
would savor the telling.

We drove a short distance on the Old Philadelphia Pike
to a grassy lane. It ran between an uncut hay field and a
tobacco patch, its plants' leaves closed for the night. At the
lane's end our headlights shone on several dozen cars
parked randomly in an apple orchard. A variety of horses,
hitched to carriages and spring wagons, were tied in the

tall grass along both sides of a rail fence, herringbone-fashion. The horses stamped wet weeds or whinnied when new wagons arrived.

Faint streaks of day shone in the east as we waded through drenched grass to the cherry trees and joined the silent wave of men, women, and children converging on a central weighing station in a clearing. We heard only the swish of plodding shoes or bare feet in the sodden morning.

By lantern light, one Kauffman brother stood beside a feed scale weighing a conglomeration of pails, kettles, and cans. Each family's containers were weighed as a unit and written on a lined tablet.

Henry K. Petersheim	3 lb.
Joel B. Beiler	6 lb.
Mary S. Stoltzfus	4$1/2$ lb.
Mark K. Stoltzfoos	8 lb.
Marvin W. Good	3 lb.
Suvilla A. Riehl	3$1/2$ lb.
Grace Kaiser	1$1/2$ lb.
Martha Weaver	5 lb.

"Hi, Doc. You have time to pick cherries?" the weightmaster teased. Raymond, like many, enjoyed the fantasy that physicians scooted from office to hospital to house calls without the interests or pleasures that others savored. That was partly true, but for me the garden and kitchen replaced golf and the hobbies enjoyed by my male associates. I liked my diversions and believed in them, yet I usually winced with some guilt when I was caught off duty or at play.

"Oh yes, my family likes cherries, too," I said, picking my two buckets from the scale. "Where do we pick?"

"John is down in the trees. He'll show you. Everybody pick clean as you go," he called.

We joined the heavy tide of pickers, dew dripping from our feet.

"Hi, Doc. Want light or dark cherries?" John Kauffman asked. "Here's a nice tree of Bings and a sturdy ladder."

In dim dawn the surge of pickers spread out under wide-armed cherry trees. We heard the sound of plump fruit hit empty buckets, then the thud of cherry on cherry.

I climbed the ladder to the tree top, where, nurtured by sunshine, the fruit seemed larger and sweeter. Also, I intended to pit a few cherries for my breakfast and I preferred to be the marksman rather than a target! Ladder pickers were less conspicuous. When I reached the top, clustered cherries were barely distinguishable from leaves. As the light improved, I could see burgundy fruit encircling me in thick clumps.

Suvilla took her buckets to a neighboring tree where boughs swept the grass. When the day brightened, her eyes occasionally met mine in amused recognition. Tomorrow!

Anna picked beneath me with the Ivan B. Zook family. Everyone picked furiously to fill pails and return home to other chores.

Day came fast and, with increasing light, the noise level swelled as the crowd recognized friends and neighbors. Only occasional words or phrases of English were spoken.

"Hi, Sam. *Wie bischt?*"

"*Mary, couldst comma? Iss baby net grank?*"

"*Vell, Susie. Wilsht du cherries canna?*"

I lost all but simple sentences amid the garbled chatter rising on all sides with the sun. Laughter and conversation filled the orchard as pail after bucket heaped beneath the trees.

In an hour we filled our buckets and stomachs. The fruit had lost its flavor. Although there would be an undertow of late arrivals most of the day, the tide had peaked. We walked back through drier grass under a clear sky. The outgoing crowd shouted and jested to the newcomers.

"No cherries left. We picked them all."

"Cherries are not good this year, sour."

We lined up, helping to find our names on the long pages.

"Well, Doc. Looks like 28 pounds."

We paid, set our buckets in the station wagon and joined the exodus.

"Cherry-picking must stir up labor," Suvilla laughed from the back seat. "My contractions are getting stronger. I'll get you breakfast; then maybe I can get some of these cherries canned."

Suvilla sped around her kitchen. She measured sugar for syrup from a hundred-pound bag. From the pantry, a shelf-lined cubicle off one end of the kitchen, she carried a blue agate canner and quart jars. After washing and draining the fruit she poked and packed it into the glass jars, poured hot syrup over the cherries, and screwed on dome lids before setting the containers in the canner of water to boil.

Our labor patient heated milk and poached eggs in it; then poured them over saltines for our breakfast. We had coffee and shoo-fly pie. The source of the name for this pie is lost. On my childhood Pennsylvania farm it was breakfast fare. Suvilla's pie was sticky and gooey on the bottom, topped by sweet fluffy crumbs. I held my breath, lifting each forkful with care, afraid I might waft away the delicate topping.

While Suvilla worked, we talked and laughed. At intervals she stopped to pant and rub her abdomen.

"Time to quit and go to bed," she announced when the last cherry was jarred. "Better call Isaiah from the barn."

If any man could be called wispy, it would be Isaiah Riehl. His beard had not grown full and heavy. Instead, below his sharp features hair stood out in meager brown tufts from a pointed chin. He was no more than five feet six inches tall and weighed about 120 pounds. He was gaunt and pale with a cough that concerned me.

He lathered and scrubbed vigorously at the kettlehouse sink, working to remove the harness oil and grit of his trade. When he strode jauntily into the bedroom, dressed in clean shirt and pants to sit beside his wife, he was the master of his house.

Isaiah spoke gently but firmly to Suvilla, never with harsh words as he guided and comforted her through the final stages of labor.

"That's it. Push now," he said. "No fuss. It'll be over soon."

Anna waited with warm blankets. I gloved and watched as a small head appeared.

"Lie still. Rest," Isaiah coached, following my signals.

A baby girl soon lay on the bed. We wrapped her in a blanket and laid her in Suvilla's arms.

"You will have to call her Cherry," Anna teased.

"An Amish Cherry?" Suvilla laughed.

Isaiah held his daughter a minute, smiled, and said nothing. Then he took a shovel and buried the placenta deep between the cabbages. We stuffed the soiled pads under the kettle and Isaiah burned them.

As we returned to New Holland and afternoon office hours, the countryside had become alive with activity. Hay-makers cut grasses to dry in the sun. Hoes and culti-vators cleaned tobacco patches. Small children played in yards, while older ones helped shell peas or picked string beans.

We saw few housewives. They must have been in their kitchens—canning cherries.

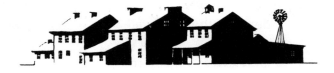

4.
Beginning

The telephone across the hall in the interns' lounge jangled like a fire alarm in the humid August air.

Quickly, I untangled my damp limbs from my bedmate's and stumbled through the semi-darkness. Lights were too risky. I could not chance getting caught in my see-through shortie by a fellow intern on the prowl at 2:00 a.m.

The ringing must stop before my male colleagues on the third floor awoke, growling complaints. As the intern on call, I would have a happier day tomorrow if I did not disturb the sleeping hive.

A street lamp at the front sidewalk tossed leafy patterns into the room, giving phantom shapes to the shabby couch and chairs.

It felt good to escape the scanty mattress. Two bodies in one hospital bed presented difficulties, even with the bed pushed against the wall. At times my companion muttered, pressed closer to the plaster, or slung an arm or leg over mine, hunting more space. Sleep was sporadic and came only if we faced the same direction. Turning over was a cooperative maneuver. I clung with stubborn persistence to the outer edge of the bed, aware even in half-sleep of the hard linoleum floor three feet below.

I stubbed a toe on the coffee table while locating the telephone. "Hello. What's up?" I asked, half-awake.

"I'll need help over here," the night intern answered. "A possible appendectomy and a labor patient just came in."

In 1950, night interns at our small hospital wrote histories and physicals, drew blood, did emergency laboratory work, and checked all labor patients (no nurse examinations permitted). We poured ether in the delivery room or scrubbed to assist the attending physician in surgery and obstetrics.

"Coming right over, Hank." I could escape the stuffy quarters for a few hours and go to the brick hospital across the drive, wander its three floors and chip ice from the hundred-pound blocks hauled daily into chests by panting ice men. Droning fans circulated medicinal air down dimly lit halls. Whispered voices of the night nurses at their knitting sedated the fervor of daytime activity like a barbiturate.

"Looks like a hot belly," Hank said when I found him in the basement laboratory hunched over a microscope counting white blood cells on the grid below the lens. He clicked off 100. "Take a squint."

"One appendectomy coming up," I agreed after listening to the patient's symptoms.

"I'll call the chief resident," Hank said.

Mike, the chief surgical resident, was responsible for all surgical patients as well as the discipline, rotating schedule, and supervision of five interns. If we erred, it put his neck in a noose.

He fit the image of a relentless demagogue. He was demanding, tyrannical, and easily given to unpredictable fits of anger. When the surgeons were unhappy, his tantrums fell on us. He was never satisfied. It seemed that no matter what I did, I—a woman—was his favorite victim.

Internships at mid-century were not required for practice in Pennsylvania and were difficult to find. I was the second woman to gain one at this Lancaster, Pennsylvania, hospital. The reputation of all female physicians seemed to rest on my shoulders. In this male-dominated profession the men seemed to believe that women wasted valuable training time if they later deserted medicine to assume household responsibilities.

The male staff treated me lightly, sure that I would quit under stress or fade into the kitchen within a few years. I resolved to prove them wrong.

Hank scrubbed for the appendectomy. I did the rectal examinations on the obstetrical patient and, during her delivery, pierced a lead-capped ether can with a safety pin to drop the ether onto a gauze mask held over her nose and mouth until she became disoriented. Her reward came with the birth of a son.

It was nearly sunrise when I climbed the stairs to my cubicle room and tossed my starched high-necked jacket and poplin skirt across the metal bureau, a chipped discard from a patient room.

My husband sprawled full width on the iron bed like a hound under a bush during a July heat wave.

"About face. Roll over, Rover," I ordered, using Chief Mike's tone.

"Okay," he grunted, bumping the wall.

I fell into the arms of young love, eager to begin my 48

hours off duty at 7:00 a.m. Husband Peter and I could resume townhunting.

"Our town must have a good highway to Lancaster in case I have to get a job in the city," Pete said.

"Must need a doctor and be a country practice," I insisted.

"You'll need a reasonable distance to the hospital, too."

"We'll want a good school system and a clean country atmosphere to raise our family."

After three months of scrutinizing towns and crossroad villages we decided upon rural New Holland, 12 miles east of Lancaster, population about 6,000.

This colonial village sat like a clucking hen above long fertile valleys of small farms, over which Amish, Mennonite, and other God-fearing families had dragged their plows for generations. New Holland, a center of buying and selling, looked right for us.

Throughout eastern Lancaster County small brooks wandered the lush pastures. Languid crossroad hamlets speckled the countryside. New Holland stretched three miles along Route 23 like a shoestring. Reared on a farm, I found the verdant area familiar. We brought parents, aunts, and uncles for their approval.

From my earliest years when I secretly mixed potions of vinegar, mustard, and pepper for my doll patients while Mother was upstairs or in the yard, being a doctor was my choice. But during my premedical years, pressured between calculus and chemistry's quantitative analysis, I became frustrated and discouraged and approached Father as he repaired a chair in the basement.

"Dad, I think I'll finish college and teach chemistry."

With measured deliberation he laid his hammer on the

workbench and glared his fiercest scowl. "What do you want to do, let some man support you all your life?" he asked with contempt.

No more said. I returned to books and laboratory. Mother, educated as a teacher but never permitted to work after marriage, smiled and said nothing.

I chafed with impatience during what seemed like endless years of structured education and blundered through mathematics, chemistry, and long afternoon laboratory sessions.

Female medical students were not taken seriously. Women on the teaching staff appeared as overly dedicated, masculine-looking frumps with few outside interests. I intended not to join them, so I kept to my own affairs with my eyes on the goal. At the end of my third year I married Peter, freshly graduated from college, and we settled in Philadelphia for my last year.

When I got an internship, we were ready to leave the grimy city. Pete folded the Murphy Bed for the last time in our third floor, two-room apartment, packed his matrimonial bags, and returned to his parents. Weekends that I did not work, he spent with me in Lancaster.

I began a year of 12- to 36-hour days for which I was paid $25.00 a month, plus room and board—if the cooks didn't close the kitchen before we got down for supper.

My first few weeks at the hospital were lonely. During free evenings I learned to operate the telephone switchboard, or fraternized with nurses as they sat at their stations, patched rubber surgical gloves for autoclaving, or cleaned intravenous tubing. Despite special solvents and rinses run through the tubing, flecks of blood still seemed to cling to the thick rubber walls.

Life improved when net-capped Elizabeth Schmook took me under her wing and explained my new world. She befriended all the interns. As a nurse's aide on the surgical floor, she handled patients with an ease that belied the 75 extra pounds on her five-foot-one frame. "Don't have a man to worry me," she always said when patients asked how she could laugh so much.

On one of my visits to her apartment I watched her rub soft dough between her palms into hot broth. Although the "rivels" in the bottom of the soup bowl never became my favorite recipe, she freely shared her Pennsylvania Dutch dishes with me, as well as information about the various Amish and Mennonite groups of Lancaster County. Schmooky would heave herself into a chrome kitchen chair and dip soup from the enamel pot into bowls. Happiness was a receptive listener.

Every week Pete heard my latest information. These people, so reserved and separate from my world, left me awe-struck. I was eager to meet them outside the hospital and see their names on my office charts. Would they accept a female physician in a culture where women are subjugated to men?

As carefully as counting blood cells on a grid, my husband and I traveled Lancaster County roads in search of our town. We wondered at buggies with fold-down tops or no tops, fascinated by the black- and gray-canvassed wagons.

How should I speak to these people? What would I say? Are they friendly or aloof? Should I address them by the conventional "Mr." and "Mrs." or by their first names?

About to leave the protective womb of institutional life, I was both eager to begin practice on my own but fearful of the unknown.

Our choosing New Holland was a serious decision. We drove through it repeatedly. In the center of town at Stauffer's Pharmacy, Plank's Plumbing, and Trimmer's Store, old tin roofs hung over the sidewalks like baseball caps. We stubbed our toes on the tilted flagstones along Main Street.

Rubinson's five-floor department store still stocked high-button shoes and rummage counters of styleless garments, purchased in large lots at fire sales in nameless cities.

We were told that the trolley tracks to Lancaster had been removed only eight years previously. Dial telephones were soon to become a reality.

We were satisfied. Our course was set. Now for a house.

"REAL ESTATE—INSURANCE Ben W. Sensenig" lettered a sign on Main Street. Here we learned the easy, off-the-cuff manner in which country folk do business. It seemed to take forever to reach a point. We discussed population, banking, the five physicians in town, and the weather.

"Where you from?" Ben asked.

"Eastern Pennsylvania."

"Why did you pick New Holland?" he pressed us. "What kinda house you lookin' for?"

Ben's desk, a filing cabinet, and two chairs crowded the sliver of space partitioned from one end of a small living room. A radio softly played religious music. In the next room a baby tottered around her playpen. We could look into a dining area and kitchen. The odor of frying onions mingled with the cloud from Ben's cigar.

Our real estate agent was gaunt with a tall and spindly spareness. He waved thin arms like wind-blown blades on a cornstalk. Tasseled brown hair topped his head. He jabbed frequently at rimless glasses, pushing them over his spiny nose. One loose lens trembled as he emphasized a sentence or swiveled his chair to hunt in files for available houses. A green and yellow Hawaiian shirt flapped like a windless sail against his body.

"Got just the place," Ben said, waving a pencil. "Three bedrooms, on Broad Street, 2,000 square feet."

"No good," I said. "We need a house on Main Street. A big one."

"Okay." He leaned over a nondescript pile of papers and picked up the phone with a cocky, I'll-fix-them air.

"A house big enough for home and office," Pete reminded him, rubbing his chin cleft.

The concept of a physician's office and home in the same building was the only one I knew. In Lancaster only specialists practiced in rooms near the hospital. At mid-century a physician was still expected to live in and be an active member of the community in which he made his living.

"Hello, Ida. Yes, this is B.W. I'm fine. You? No, I didn't hear about that." He tilted his chair against the wall. "Do you know if Luke Sauder is home? Guess his house is still for sale. Ring him up, please."

My wooden chair was hard. Had we found the right agent?

Pete wiped his wire-framed glasses, rubbed boyish apple cheeks, brushed a hand over thinning brown hair.

"You want a big house. Luke's house should be big enough," Ben said critically. "Not cheap, though." He seemed to discern our thin pocketbooks. "A woman doctor in New Holland." He shook his head and smiled.

"We'll take a look," I said, undaunted. Renting never

occurred to us. Our roots were to be planted deep and permanently.

"Luke's place is an old farmhouse on half an acre, 10 rooms, brick," Ben said.

"Good," we agreed.

"You young folks have financing?"

"No. We'll get a mortgage, of course."

If I thought Ben's lens quivered when I had said "woman doctor," it certainly shook when two young strangers expected to buy a house without funds. He smiled civilly and rose to shake Pete's hand and dismiss the time-wasters.

"Luke's wife is home. She'll show you the house," Ben said. "Stop back if I can help again."

The Sauder house at 561 West Main Street, built in 1865, was the home for us. I knew it instantly. My fantasy of again living in an old farmhouse would be realized. She was a queen, white-painted brick, enthroned on grassy banks four feet above street level, and looking down on smaller neighbors through blue-shuttered windows. Two giant elms shaded her west porches and walls.

We walked under a twisted and hollow Kiefer pear tree to the east porch and kitchen door. Hard pears still clung to the high branches and littered the ground. Marigolds, petunias, and asters girdled the house. A long rose bed edged the macadam drive to the street.

Martha Sauder greeted us at the old wooden screen door. She led us through a large living room opening onto the front porch by two doors.

"This big room, the bedroom, and bath next to it are just what I need for office space," I murmured to Pete.

"We're building a new house on the dirt street behind

Main," Martha said, showing us two upstairs bedrooms and a bath. "We rent out a four-room apartment on the second floor."

"Income," Pete said. "And living space for us, too."

"What's that shed hanging onto the back of the house?" I asked.

"The old milk house," Martha said. "We tore the barn away last year." She pointed to an arbor where a few last leaves fluttered in the October air. "You'll get good grapes."

"Don't lean against the garage," I whispered to Peter.

The flimsy frame building listed decidedly southward. The lawn mower and assorted stacked boxes seemed to support the drunken shack.

Lace curtains in the house next door fluttered perceptibly as we examined a gnarled apple tree.

"Good harvest apples—make good sauce," Martha said. "That little block building out back is the old egg shed. The apartment building on Broad Street is the remodeled chicken house. With Luke farming, he didn't get drafted during the war."

"It's not chickens at those windows," I said, as other curtains moved.

We lifted wooden porch doors and descended stone steps to inspect three dirt cellars.

"There's a thousand-gallon tank buried in the yard and a 500 one down here," Martha said. "We paid 16 cents a gallon last winter for oil."

We should have been forewarned when we saw the monster, a converted coal furnace and the cellar's focal point. Its octopus arms reached out in all directions.

When I saw the big flower boxes on the front lawn I envisioned a blast of summer color onto Main Street. Martha forgot to tell us about the gigantic tree stumps they obscured.

We trampled through thick grass and never estimated the hours required to mow it.

The sunny day we visited, no driving east rain came through the bricks and ran down the inside wall. Nor did a blizzard blow snow around rattling window sash and pile flakes onto the deep sills.

"We can push some paste behind the loose wallpaper," Pete said. "But I'll have to give the outside a paint job soon. It looks like a long way up to those attic eaves."

Ben got a phone call two days later. "We'll take the Sauder house," I said.

The price of $18,500 was gargantuan for our empty pockets. We depended on a government housing loan for veterans. The inspector probed and tapped every wall and floor from attic to cellar. He remarked that the beautiful pine boards had no subflooring and the plaster had been applied directly to brick walls. Application denied. We appealed. Then, considering the age of the house, we were granted an exception.

The final storm appeared the fiercest. In order to meet government requirements at the bank, we needed one-third of the purchase price as down payment. It could not be borrowed. They might as well have asked for all of it. Our plans washed away on a flood of the impossible.

My parents rescued us. A four percent mortgage and the big house on Main Street were ours. We sailed smoother waters.

In February Pete began work in the office of New Holland Machine Company. Until the end of my intern commitment on July first, I spent weekends and days off in our new home.

We bought the kitchen stove from Martha, ate at a cast-off attic table, and sat on flimsy, bargain-priced, card-table chairs. A borrowed pickup transported an antique bedroom suite and a refrigerator to complete our furnishings.

Proudly, we walked through the hollow house, spending money years in advance. Our footsteps echoed through the empty rooms. We brushed snow off winter window sills, chinked cracks with rags, and pasted curling wallpaper.

At last we slept in our own house, in a queen-sized bed. The street light at the curb threw shadows into the bedroom. I could reach onto the table beside my pillow and find the telephone.

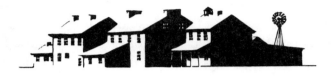

5.
Naomi's Birthing

"Impossible," I said, half to myself and half to Naomi Glick. Naomi had just finished her final prenatal visit and, shifting in the chair beside my desk, did not rise to leave.

"No, I haven't told Simon yet," she repeated. Slender fingers, tanned from work in field and garden, picked nervously at threads escaping seams on the large green satchel on her lap. Its fabric was probably left over from an upholstered chair or couch at home. The amber plastic handles were sold from racks at Rubinson's Store in New Holland.

"Haven't told him?" I repeated.

"I didn't know what he'd say." Naomi sighed and leaned against the leather chair, relieved to have finally told me. Clear brown eyes searched my face for a response.

"Not told him. How can he miss it?" I nearly shouted. With Naomi almost at term with her fifth baby, how could Simon not know, when the bulge that sagged behind her apron proclaimed "baby" to the world. Instinctively, I ran a hand over my own expanded abdomen.

Simon knew. He was a caring man. Whenever I saw him in town or about the farm, two or three of his boys rode beside him in the wagon or shadowed him as he worked.

"No, I mean about you," Naomi laughed, showing fine white teeth. Her round face, tanned and satin smooth, flushed like a ripe peach at mentioning my pregnancy.

"Don't worry about me. You'll beat me by at least six weeks," I predicted with confidence, touching my mounded dress.

I squirmed under the heat and pressure of the elastic stockings hanging from my shoulders by an ingenious strap arrangement. Certainly the contraption was designed by a man. No woman would harness another, even for a day, in such a web. Naomi surely must suffer beneath the weight and color of her black clothing.

The July heat was intensified by Naomi's black long-sleeved dress, black cape, and apron. Simon's mother had died in May. Naomi would wear black everywhere for a year.

Air conditioning was virtually unknown in 1953 except in a few commercial buildings. Electric fans were the most one could expect. People talked about the heat, worried about polio, and awaited September with its cooler days.

"I was afraid Simon would make me change doctors," Naomi continued, wiping her wet brow and rimless glasses on a man's white handkerchief. Her cheeks dimpled. "I'm relieved our dates won't conflict," she said. Her abdomen was much larger and more obvious than mine.

Amish women do not sew special maternity dresses, I was told. "We make our dresses and aprons generous enough to keep letting the waistline's straight pins out as we expand." When an Amish mother nurses her baby she removes the straight pins from her dress, sticks them into her cape where they will not scratch the baby, and separates the dress beneath her cape, exposing her breast to the baby. It is a maneuver so discreet that few people in a busy room notice the feeding.

My pregnancy, six weeks from term, stretched the only remaining dress I could close. Weekends I submitted to tent-like maternity clothes. This last frock of green and white plaid spanned my belly. Its belt, having passed its final hole, hung abandoned in the closet. A temperamental snap at the waistline popped if I overate, stooped, or laughed.

I had tried to hide my pregnancy from patients as long as possible, worried about their loyalty. Country people appeared to accept pregnancy almost as they did eating or sleeping. But how would they feel about a gravid doctor? Would men patients go elsewhere? I no longer had a secret.

My practice did not seem to diminish. I never discussed the pregnancy. Business was as usual.

"When will you tell Simon?" I asked, comparing her garden-stained hands, devoid of jewelry, to my large ones wearing wedding band, diamond, and watch.

"Maybe today." Her brown eyes avoided mine, her face anxious.

"Be sure to call for another appointment if you go overtime," I said.

Naomi extracted a pocket watch from her cavernous bag. "I have to walk downtown to meet Simon. He dropped me off here, then tied our team at Kauffman's Hardware." She scooped a bottle of vitamins from the desk. "I think everything will be okay."

During the early years of my practice I was also the receptionist and nurse. I walked with Naomi through the waiting room to the front door. At the moment there was no next patient to see. From the window I watched Naomi walk down Main Street until she disappeared at Hollinger's Esso Station. Would I see her again?

From childhood I had two goals in life: first, a medical career, and then children. In that order. Plans called for their peaceful coexistence. After two years of general practice I saw increasing signs of career success. Now I could feel my baby snuggled in my arms, hear its garbled mutterings, smell Johnson's powder.

Having children surely would not interfere with my career. Four years of marriage seemed a long wait to have a baby. I vowed not to allow family to conflict with profession.

Naomi was the first hint of trouble. I must be patient, wait for Simon's call when labor began. Would he call? Would he give approval for the new woman doctor, now pregnant, to deliver his wife? Was it my professional abilities he doubted? My male peers had predicted that a woman could not succeed in the country. Could they have been right? I wondered, would my having a family make a difference?

A good rapport and mutual bond existed between Naomi and me. Every day I thought of her and waited. It seemed as if my professional future hung on the little woman from Dry Hill who had chosen me to deliver her baby, but feared to tell her husband that her doctor, too, was "in the family way."

Each day dragged and my fear of abandonment grew. The morning newspaper did not print a birth for Simon and Naomi Glick, but after 10 days I was certain that I had been traded for a more responsible male physician. Disappointed, I resolved to forget her.

When or how Naomi told Simon about her pregnant doctor I never knew. I didn't ask. Twelve days after the office visit Simon called from a neighbor's telephone. His wife was in labor, soon to deliver at home.

My station wagon splashed through summer showers as it climbed Heim's Hill and through the sultry heat of late July. The air was heavy with moisture, and I felt like a fish gulping for breath. Intense summer clung to every bush and blade. It penetrated the thickest house walls. Oppressive humid air made nights as miserable as days. With no relief in sight for eastern Pennsylvania, I concluded that pregnancy was no summer picnic.

Naomi's burden was soon to be delivered. She had children and a husband with whom to share her days. My husband was 3,000 miles away guiding Boy Scouts to a National Jamboree in California. It made me uneasy, and I looked forward to his return the next week.

As I drove down the south slope, I wondered how Simon would greet me. He would not mention my pregnancy. Within Amish families there is sharp teasing. Sisters and sisters-in-law accuse each other of pregnancies at every additional pound of weight, trying to "worm out" secrets. Husbands gibe each other when they group for gossip after church or at family gatherings. I was a stranger. Nothing would be said.

The source of the name "Dry Hill" remains a mystery. The evening I turned into Glick's homestead, their lane's gravel tracks were awash with the recent showers. Fields of head-high corn pressed the lane to its edges. Each spiked blade of deep green dripped water. Majestic rows of arched leaves created endless vaults in a Gothic cathedral. In the gentle evening light no breeze rustled the cornstalk pillars that swallowed the lane near the horizon.

In a clearing, Glick's great white barn, numerous out-buildings, and the sprawling brick farmhouse seemed an island in an emerald ocean.

As I left the car and turned to pick up my bag, the dress snap parted. This was no time to be frivolous. Quickly, I closed it and sucked in my breath, vowing to put the green plaid away tomorrow.

I stepped along a flagstone walk between whitewashed arbors hanging full with vines and half-grown chartreuse grapes in thick clusters. My black bag unbalanced the weight beneath the snap. I held the dress tightly.

Unsmiling, Simon met me at a glass-enclosed porch outside the kitchen. He thrust a leg forward and held open the wooden screen door. His great stubby toes looked as if they had not seen shoes since he discarded them when the horse chestnuts bloomed last spring. One middle toe was swathed in laminated bandaids.

"Good evening," he said politely, leading the way through a long kitchen. Squeezing past him in the doorway, I imagined I was being appraised, as if he were assessing the value of a new cow in the barn.

Simon filled his broadfalls well. Several layers of patch-es contrasted new black with washed-out gray. Shrunken by many Monday launderings, they rose to heavy calves. A faded lavender shirt, rolled above the elbows, exposed sun-bronzed arms thick as a city man's thighs. His heavy jowls were hidden by a dark beard that extended ear to ear and lay on his chest like a forkful of hay. He carried a razor in one hand and flecks of shaving cream spotted his upper lip and face above the untrimmed beard.

"Hot night," I said, looking for any signal of approval, a smile or twinkle in the black-brown eyes. I saw none.

"Yes, it is," he said flatly. He laid the razor on the hand sink and toweled his face. "Naomi's in the bedroom." He waved a burly hand toward the far part of the kitchen, sat down in a swivel chair at the end of the long table, and picked up the morning paper.

I heard women's voices in the bedroom conversing in Pennsylvania Dutch. "Good evening, Doctor." A dumpy little woman padded across the bedroom, smiled and shook my hand. "I'm Mary Stoltzfoos from Churchtown. Thought maybe you could use some help." She wore a plain black cape and apron and a brightly colored dress with short sleeves. Her thick legs and feet were bare. From her white hair, beneath a white organdy cap, I estimated her age between 50 and 60. Evening half-light hid many wrinkles in her pleasant face.

"Naomi says your time is soon here. How old are you?" Naomi's mother quizzed. "What does your husband work? Out in California, eh? He'd better not stay too long. Works for New Holland Machine Company? I thought you would be older. I hope your man gets home soon," she chuckled, eyeing me from my middle, then up, down, and back again.

"I'm glad for a granny to help," I said, thinking how Mary came directly to a point. I unpacked my bag, resolved to say and do everything with caution.

It was common policy, particularly during my earlier years of practice, to have a mother, aunt, or any older married woman act as "granny" during a delivery. They gathered linens, dressed the baby, and stayed after the birth until the self-trained, unmarried Amish nurse could be "fetched." These nurses made their livelihood traveling from one new mother to another, acting as nurse and surrogate mother for the household.

"I never helped a woman doctor before," Mary said, her broad face breaking into a grin. "Guess it isn't different than helping men doctors. Seems funny not to have a man around a time like this." She clucked, shaking her head.

Finally I knew why Naomi feared that Simon would not approve of me, why Simon had been cool and unsmiling. He was unsure, ill at ease, and embarrassed with a strange woman, particularly a pregnant one, in the house during an intimate situation.

Mary gave me approval with her smile and good humor. Now for the delivery. While Simon sat silently behind his newspaper, Mary and I attended the patient.

Simon rose occasionally from his chair to swat flies with a red swatter imprinted "KING'S HARNESS SHOP—Intercourse, PA." He walked to the doorway and watched the bedroom activities, saying little. His fly-swatting excursions became more frequent, conversations longer.

We waited 90 minutes for the birth. Mary ambled about the bedroom, picking and choosing baby clothes from a drawer. She laid an old blanket on the bed in which to wrap the new baby, brought a cookie sheet and kitchen scales from the pantry to weigh the newborn, tore an old sheet into rags for cleaning mother and child.

When we could no longer see in the dusky room, Simon lit a pressure lamp and hung it from a ceiling hook above the footboard. Heat from the hissing lantern added discomfort to the muggy room.

Outside, the night seethed with an arpeggio of crickets. Little moved in the stagnant air. A cow bawled in a meadow. Dogs barked in the distance; others answered.

Our clothing hung damp and stuck to our bodies. No breeze moved the green window shades pulled against varnished sills in case someone would drive in the lane. I stopped caring about my impossible snap. A slit of white underwear herniated through the gap.

Naomi labored and perspired on the bed. At times she sat up to cool her heated back. Mary folded cold wet washcloths against her neck and chest and wiped her arms and face with them.

Mary removed her black cape and apron, folded them over a chair back, and stored their straight pins in the wide apron belt. She removed the top pin from her dress, untied her stiff cap strings, and pinned them behind her neck. Every few minutes she mopped her beaded brow with an immense man's handkerchief, pulling it from her pocket with a flourish. She fanned Naomi with a sheet of old newspaper folded into quarters.

As often as possible I leaned near enough to my patient to catch a momentary supply of the cooling draft. I wondered what circumstances would surround my delivery. Mother lived miles away from New Holland, and in those years mothers and husbands were not allowed in hospital delivery areas. They were condemned to long anxious hours in stuffy waiting rooms. My husband could not sit in the next room, ready to come to my side if I wanted him or needed him.How many hours would I be in labor, every complaint and action witnessed by doctors and nurses I knew well? Would I be as relaxed, calm, and quiet as Naomi? Would the weather be as hot and unbearable as this night?

While Mary fanned and mopped and wiped she educated me on the births of her 14 children, their names, and present ages. I followed the family genealogy from a framed fraktur on the wall. It was neatly lettered and decorated with pink and red roses. She spoke proudly of 56 grandchildren, four unmarried children at home, one daughter killed in a buggy-auto accident, and a son lost to a childhood case of typhoid. Tortuous leg and foot veins, the size of pencils, mapped her numerous pregnancies.

My elastic stockings became heavier and hotter as Naomi labored. I longed for my delivery day. I folded a paper and fanned my face and neck, aching to go home, undress, and relax.

Discomfort seemed to urge Naomi along. Her delivery was noiseless, calm, not difficult. Would I behave as well? Could I be without whimper or complaint? She set a good example.

If I could only have known that on a hot night like Naomi's, Peter and I would scarcely make it to the hospital on time and that the doctor would barely arrive to deliver our daughter, I would have worried instead about speed.

Simon came into the bedroom to watch the delivery. "It will soon be over now, Nomi," he said, standing by her head. "Do what the doctor tells you."

In the '50s there were no practiced breathing exercises, no controlled relaxation, no instructed husband involvement. Most women at home were stoic, at ease, self-controlled. A few wanted anesthetic whiffs of the ether or trilene that I carried in my bag.

"You're doing fine without any shot or something to breathe," Mary said as the birth neared. "The baby's nearly here."

"It's a girl, Nomi. We finally have a girl," Simon said, hoarsely, when the baby lay on the bed.

"A girl at last. A girl. Thank you. Thank you. Thank you." Naomi repeated at least three times. "And it took a woman doctor to do it!"

I felt proud and exhilarated, as if I was responsible for the first Glick daughter.

"Hope I'll know how to care for a girl," Naomi beamed. "It was great to have a woman doctor. I'll always want a woman now." She raised onto an elbow to watch her mother bathe and dress her fifty-seventh grandchild.

Mary wrapped the baby and covered it in an infant crib. We lifted the crib's foot end onto a chair. In that era, babies got nothing to eat for 12 hours.

Naomi needed no sutures, fortunately for me, since bending over a bed was difficult for this doctor. Resting in a clean bed, Naomi beamed satisfaction, triumph.

The household would be in Mary's care until morning when Simon could fetch nurse Barbara Zook. Mary and Naomi smiled at each other, smiled at me. We had shared, become friends. Even Simon smiled when he passed in and out of the bedroom on errands. He stopped each time at the crib to admire his daughter, vigorously sucking her fist.

"Guess we'll have to have you come again if we want another girl," Simon laughed.

I drove home from Dry Hill drenched in victory.

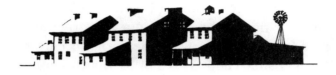

6.
Barks and Bites

One last postnatal call to an Amish family near Cattail Crossing south of New Holland and I could go home and shower the day's heat and dust down the drain.

Mid-August humidity hung over the eastern seaboard like one big cloud. Everyone gulped the wet air and complained about the heat and sleepless nights.

The day so far had been as predictable as the plot of a Sunday school Christmas pageant. Patients during morning office hours had seemed difficult to please and their complaints not easily satisfied. "Doctor, why?" and "Doctor, when?" and "Doctor, could you?"

I was glad when the last patient left at noon, and I started afternoon house calls. Air blowing through the open car windows relieved some of my discomfort. An eighth month bulge beneath my dress did not improve the day. This third summer of pregnancy was as novel as eggs to an old setting hen.

When I slowed onto Noah R. Blank's lane, a dirty flag of

dust billowed in the air. It clung to the head-high corn planted to the edge of the dusty tracks. Corn changed to a field of tobacco. Noah and seven or eight barefooted children sweated in its harvest. They stopped to wave.

When I stepped onto the graveled lane near the yard fence that set the house apart from the drive and barn, Shep flew from the shadow of the corncrib barking furiously. I stood still. The massive St. Bernard-shepherd mix bolted across the barnyard with undisputed malice. Three gulps would devour me.

Most farmers kept biting dogs tied, their purpose to ward off thieves and arsonists who victimized tinder-dry unguarded barns. Shep probably was harmless, but his attitude was as friendly as a fox treed by a pack of hounds. I would handle him.

"Get to the barn you good-for-nothing bum," I commanded, taking a step toward galloping Goliath.

He belonged to the 90 percent bluff group. My attacker stopped and shook his hairy head, questioning my authority.

"I mean it. Get out!" I shouted, stamping a foot.

It was humorous to see him tuck his tail between his legs and sulk to the barn. Near the corner of the milkhouse he turned to see if I still meant business. I doubt if he understood English, but my tone was unmistakable. He lumbered out of sight.

I left the protection of my car and opened the wire gate into the yard and long concrete walk stretching to the house several hundred yards away. The sprawling brick and frame farmhouse seemed to slumber in beds of geraniums, asters, and marigolds. As usual in hot weather, the upstairs shutters were closed against the sun. The less exposed bricks behind the shutters were a darker shade. The house had closed its eyes for a nap; its roof capped the brow.

With a full skirt flapping around my legs and my black bag swaying with each step, I had plodded about a quarter of the distance to the washhouse door when the new attack came.

From under the cooler earthen recess of the front porch steps, two small dogs flew across the lawn with the fury of a tropical hurricane.

These dogs meant business. No bluffing here. I looked for help. The house slept on, did not open an eye. Quiet. Sadie, Noah's wife, was confined with her new baby. Noah and the children were in the tobacco field.

Where were these dogs yesterday when I attended the birthing? They had probably been in the *dawdy* end of the house with Grandmother and the children. I was taken off guard by this canine assault and too clumsy and slow to outrun it.

Peggy, a rat terrier, ran in the lead. Her white body, splotched irregularly with brown, shook with bark and wrath. Between white pyramid ears a capricious flow of black covered one eye like a wink. She was an ornery terror, ready to add to her list of milkmen and deliverymen— doctor.

Behind Peggy raced half a handful of black Chihuahua. She covered her cohort's rear flank, snapping and yapping. Pepper, a small tornado on toothpick legs, belonged to Mommy Blank in the frame house annex called the *dawdy haus.*

This sport was not new to this pair. I stopped. The dogs jumped, barked, and snarled. They lunged, retreated, and lunged again. When I walked forward they attacked closer. The louder I shouted the fiercer they became. My bag became a shield.

No rescue in sight. I inched along the walk. Finally the beasts allowed me to pass. I relaxed. They stopped barking, became quiet, slunk toward the barn. Safe.

Then it happened.

From behind me, Peggy jumped to her quarry. Teeth clamped my right ankle and held fast. I swung my leg forward but she held tight. At the height of my forward kick, Peggy released her grip, landed on the walk with a yip, scrambled to her feet, and began barking again. Blood oozed through my elastic stocking. My leg burned.

"*Geh veck! Geh naus!*" baby nurse Annie Petersheim shouted from the front porch. The barking dogs and my shouting had ended nap time. She ran to my rescue.

"Come in here. Let's take a look at your leg. Better doctor you up," Annie insisted, shooing the dogs as she came down the walk.

My enemies reluctantly withdrew to their lair under the steps. But Peggy would not forget the taste of my blood. Her eyes glinted triumph.

The situation between Peggy and me deteriorated. Winter or summer she always lay in wait when I stepped inside the yard fence. Whenever Noah expected me, he penned my adversary in the washhouse, and I used the kitchen door at the front of the house. The dog would bark and throw herself against the door into the kitchen until I left. I savored each visit with a tinge of victory.

A cold January day several years later, Noah called me to deliver Sadie. It was also a stork race. Noah hurried me up the snowy walk and through the washhouse. Without time to remove my coat, I caught the wiggling, squalling, fourteenth Blank baby in ungloved hands.

In the scurry of postpartum care, I walked between bedroom and kitchen many times. The unexpected rush of the delivery allowed me no time to think of Peggy. In the absence of children and dogs, I assumed her to be with Mommy Blank. Other than an occasional whimper from the newborn, the only noise was the whine of wind in the stovepipe.

As I picked up my coat and black bag, I passed the hot coal range. A streak of wild fury burst from under the stove. Instinctively I dropped the bag between the raging dog and my legs. Peggy struck the satchel headfirst. She backed off, snarling and barking.

"*Geh naus! Geh veck!*" Noah shouted, surprised, too. He picked the dog up by the nape of her neck and held her against his lavender shirt where she struggled and snapped, a frenzied demon.

"Hold her until I leave," I said, speeding a retreat.

"I forgot about the dog," Noah apologized, smiling and stroking his beard in feigned concern. He could not hide his amusement at my fear of one little dog. "I'm surprised she laid quiet this long. Guess she wouldn't leave her babies."

Noah held the distraught Peggy while he groped under the stove and withdrew a Campbell's Tomato Soup box. Four sightless puppies of muddled white, jet, and cocoa, squirmed like hairless mice in a pink flannel petticoat bed.

"Want a puppy for your children?" he teased.

"No, we have a little black dog," I said, wanting none of feisty Peggy's offsprings.

"Their eyes will open Friday when they're 10 days old," Noah said, stroking Peggy gently with a broad hand stained brown from days of tobacco stripping. "Ready for adoption in another five weeks," he said, resting a thumb under his suspenders.

"The little mother would never agree with your gift."

My assailant would not be pacified. I was glad that she could not escape Noah's firm grip but also pitied the protective instinct that enraged her. For no amount of compassion would I ask Noah to release her before I closed the kitchen door behind me.

It was I who finally ended Peggy's pugnacious life. I remember it with guilt and remorse. I never intended to injure the cyclone of flying legs and snapping jaws. It is still not clear to me if the Blanks understood or forgot it. There was no triumph.

February that year had been a month of sustained cold and intermittent blizzards. The back roads were no sooner passable when another storm dumped fresh snow onto the already plowed one-way paths.

Roads were single lanes in most places. Automobiles ran like trolleys in the deep ice ruts. Once caught in a frozen ice furrow, a vehicle had no opportunity to turn out until it reached a wider cleared space.

The Cattail Road was no different. My studded tires were hopelessly ineffectual as the station wagon moved slowly between snowbanks. Braking meant skidding into a snowpile or ditch.

As I neared the Noah Blank farm, I saw Noah and several children riding a bobsled full of corn fodder. A team of sorrel horses pulled them from the field onto the road and toward the barn. Peggy and Shep trotted along on the bank across the road.

I slowed. Noah waved and pulled onto a wide place. I

crawled past, car window open. One of the children called to Peggy. She obeyed in a flash. My wheels caught her in the frozen track. She died instantly. The station wagon slid to a stop and I backed to the sleigh.

The Amishman said nothing. He descended slowly from the load of fodder, picked up the limp body, and tossed it onto the snow in the cornfield.

"We want her collar. Get her collar," several children shouted. It was a small token by which to remember the fiery pet that had shared their snacks, the kitchen couch, and her puppies. Sadfaced children sat on the load of dry cornstalks. The younger ones stifled tears.

Noah quietly climbed the snowbank to the lifeless dog, unbuckled her collar, and returned to the sleigh. He handed the collar to the children, picked up the reins in his gloved hands.

"I'm sorry," I said. "She jumped in front of my wheels."

"Yes, we saw it," Noah said. He did not smile.

I watched the sleigh full of grief pull toward the barn.

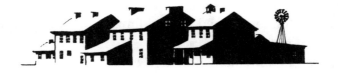

7.
Ducky

The old saying, "You get what you pay for," suited our supper entree one spring evening. Receiving a right-off-the-farm gift of food was not unusual when the rural medical practice I conducted was among generous Amish and Mennonites. Had Sarah Riehl known about her donation she might have replaced it.

Mary Stoltzfus was the first donor of the day. "Good afternoon, Doctor," she said from her seat on the low concrete wall of the porch fronting my office. In one hand she held a needle threaded with gray darning cotton, the other fist stuffed inside a black sock. "I'm early for my appointment," she said, removing a small scissors from between her teeth. "I finished shopping at Rubinson's Store and came up here to each lunch and sit in the sun." She thrust a sandwich bag and the mending into a homemade tapestry handbag and pulled out a brown paper sack. "I brought you something. Can you use these?"

"Yes, we love strawberries," I answered, downing one in

two bites. They were gigantic, brilliant red, and chin-wiping juicy. "Thank you." It was difficult to speak with too much berry in my mouth. "How much are they?"

Mary assumed the happy look of one whose time in the hot sun and backbreaking effort had been worthwhile. She gathered her packages and black bonnet and moved toward the waiting room. "I gave you those, but if you can use any more I have 10 boxes in the market wagon for sale."

"I'll buy four," I said, knowing a purchase was expected. She would either sell the rest from my waiting room or knock on neighbors' doors.

Mary adjusted her white Amish cap and trotted to the backyard where her horse stood patiently at the hitching rail.

Later, Sadie Beiler unceremoniously plopped a plastic bread bag of sugar peas on my desk. With thanks and admiration, I accepted her gift. She had none to sell, and I would have had no extra time that day to string them. I was glad sugar peas did not need shelling.

I did not barter services. Gifts were generous extras given in sincere appreciation for professional services. My family accepted them greedily. Patients happily shared their excesses. June was a month of liberal harvests.

It was not unusual to leave a country house call with a dozen eggs, a fresh loaf of bread, or a bag of raisin-dotted cookies. If the family had hosted church that Sunday, I might even receive another coveted prize, a snitz pie made with dried apples that had been cooked and spiced.

Mary's and Sadie's were not the only gifts. When afternoon office hours were finished I admired the 10 boxes of strawberries, three bags of sugar peas, and a quart of shelled hull peas, two plastic bags of cut leaf lettuce, a bundle of radishes, and one of green onions, all on the kitchen counter. Anything extra went into the big freezer in the garage.

At Christmas season the counter was often full of cookies. The children fought for favorites, usually the filled ones or chocolate chips.

As I contemplated the generosity of my patients and juggled boxes for refrigerator space, our older son came into the kitchen.

He snatched two strawberries. "What's for supper?" he asked, with the eagerness of 14 and the authority of his father. Waiting until I dove again into the refrigerator, he committed the kitchen sin and lifted each pot lid.

"Peas and new potatoes," I answered, watching Keith move over the pans.

"No, what's the meat?" he persisted.

"Duck. Sarah Riehl brought me a duck yesterday. It's in the oven. Keep the door shut. Wait until supper."

Sarah had been as proud as a child receiving praise from her favorite teacher when she handed me the duck. All the finest feathers had been removed, the hairs meticulously singed, and the bird carefully dressed before she wrapped it in plastic and a bag. She sensed I had never received a duck before. The bird offering lay plump and beautiful between us on my desk. She had given me a great gift. Her eyes were bright and happy as I thanked her.

"What's for supper?" My husband also sinned, lifting each lid as he asked his daily question.

"Nothing if you don't leave the lids on the kettles and the oven door closed. I put a duck in there several hours ago."

At supper the unusual stance of the fowl on the platter I

set before Peter did not impress me as abnormal until he set a carving knife against a leg and bore down. Nothing changed. Those stiff brown legs should have been soft and limp, falling against a tender breast. Instead, two hard drumsticks jutted upright like cannons aimed for action.

Again my husband brought his knife across the duck. Then a final try. "You forgot to turn on the oven," he laughed.

I thought I saw the bird shudder on knife contact. "No I didn't. We'll eat it another day. How about scrambled eggs?" I snatched the rigor-mortised duck from the table and got out the frying pan.

Sarah intended for us to eat that duck. I wondered how many years it had waddled through her meadow and swam on the Riehl pond. Had it been caught due to faltering old age? I did feel that I had earned the duck when I sat most of a night in Sarah's kitchen while she labored to deliver a 10-pound baby boy.

The determination to eat my benefits increased. Before evening office hours I popped the resistant bird into a pot with an onion. It simmered more than three hours. Sarah had chased, captured, plucked, and cleaned that duck, and then had given it to me. We would eat it.

When I lifted the pot lid at 10 o'clock, two rigid drumsticks pointed ceilingward. The onion dropped submissively between them. A knife still bounced off the rubbery meat.

I gave up the contest for that day, but I was not defeated. Sarah had given us the duck to eat.

The next afternoon while redressing an injured hand for patient Nancy Zook she wrinkled her nose and sniffed. "What do I smell in your office today?"

"Ssst! Ssst! Ssst!" answered the steaming autoclave at maximum heat and pressure.

"Quiet," I whispered, hoping the safety valve was good.

Later Keith hovered over the pot lids. "What's for supper?"

"Duck," I murmured. I did not look at him.

"Again. The same one?" he snickered and waited to inspect the kettles when I turned toward the sink.

"It's cooked this time. No duck will get the best of me," I said.

"Are you sure?" Peter called from the dining room. "Last night it was still tough. How did you subdue the critter?"

From an aluminum foil package, tumbled a shapeless nondescript brown mass of hot meat and bones onto a waiting platter.

"Persistence," I called victoriously.

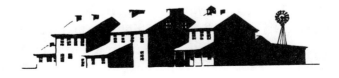

8.
God's a Woman

Emmanuel Beiler could not speak English, but at school he explained in his language that God had been to his house and left something there. Mom and Pop had told him it was so.

His father had phoned at 6:30 a.m. "Priscilla will 'be needing you' sometime today, but not right away," Daniel predicted.

"Okay for me to go to church?" I asked, irritated at being awakened early on a Sunday. He had probably been up for hours, had finished milking and perhaps his breakfast. Why shouldn't everyone be up?

"Yes, go. She's only started. I guess we won't need you 'til toward evening. Just wanted to let you know in plenty of time, like it says on the paper you gave us."

I had fed my family lunch and bedded the younger children for a nap when Daniel called again at one-thirty.

"Guess you better come soon. No hurry, though," he said.

Intermittent ice patches glazing highways and lanes made a silly jest of "hurry." Roadside trees flailed their naked limbs fitfully in a biting wind, seducing travelers into dirty snowbanks thrown up by plows after a late February blizzard. Highways had been closed for several days. In shaded places, between high banks or in woods, ice ruts gripped the car like iron rails hugging a train.

Ten days of milk and feed trucks had opened Beiler's gravel lane. The barnyard was covered with half-frozen snow tracks. I remembered to park on a level dry place near the yard fence, so as not to become trapped on an icy hill when the sun went down and temperatures dropped. Stories had spread about the several times I was pulled from mucky or iced barnyards by teams of mules or horses.

Beiler's rambling home, like most Lancaster County farmhouses, was built with the ground floor for family activities, a second story for bedrooms, an attic for storage, and a cellar for canned goods. Occasionally, if the house was built into a hill, the basement was utilized for Monday washing and summer work. At most farms the wash-house, or kettlehouse, with its great kettle set into a brick fire pit, seemed tacked on later. In the iron kettle house-wives heated Monday wash water, cooked meat during winter butchering, and often canned summer produce.

A long porch with two paneled doors and several windows usually spanned the house front. Traditionally one door opened into the parlor, the other into the kitchen. A long slate roof covered the porch of my childhood home, but many of these were roofed by upper floors or a smaller open porch with wooden balustrades. The housewife aired bedding or hung rainy day wash on the upstairs porches. In summer the lower porch was furnished with assorted rocking chairs, a metal glider, or swing hung from screeching chains.

Like many Amish families, the Beilers had enclosed part of their porch as an extension of the kitchen, using a series of glass windows. On broad shelves, on tables, and from hooks, the women created a greenhouse of geraniums, ferns, and African violets. Spring seedlings germinated and grew in plum boxes and tomato cans on sun porches until ready for the garden.

Variations in farmhouses were not only in the porches. Their floor plans roughly followed an I, L, T, or U depending upon how many pieces and patches had been added. Often an entire home, called the *dawdy haus,* was annexed for aging parents. The number and size of the additions reflected family needs and pressure from increasing population.

Noble farmhouses of brick, frame, or stone splotched the countryside, usually shaded by aged maples, oaks, or elms and surrounded by a yard fence. A pack of mongrel dogs staunchly defended farm territories.

I was glad the Beiler dogs were penned in the barn as I picked my way over watery ice patches on the salted walk.

Daniel met me at the kettlehouse door. He was dressed in Sunday's white shirt, black pants, and vest. Wind lashed the house, lifted his black bangs and ear-lobe length hair. His brown eyes squinted until they teared. He clutched his rusty beard with one hand and the doorknob with the other.

"No rush. Priscilla has some time yet," he said, taking a bandanna handkerchief to his long thin nose.

An assortment of boots and galoshes identified the household members as a woman, a man, a toddler, and child. An old cupboard at refrigerator temperature held puddings, jellos, and leftover foods. Pies and cakes loaded several shelves. Coleman lanterns, filled and ready for evening milking, sat on the wooden lid of the great iron kettle.

I stomped my boots on the concrete floor and followed Dan's long stride, glad to enter the warm kitchen. There was an empty wall hook behind the Warm Morning space heater for my coat.

"Hi, Grace," Priscilla said, with a smile that accentuated her high cheek bones. "A real March day." Sunday being a day of rest, she paced the room or entertained the children.

The room seemed warmer when Priscilla addressed me by first name, and I thought with sympathy of my city peers who would not tolerate or understand this informality.

"Priscilla thinks it could go several hours yet," Dan said combing his beard. "But . . . it might go fast like the last time, too."

In addition to the kettlehouse door, two others led from the kitchen. The door to the unheated parlor was closed. The door to Dan's and Priscilla's bedroom, warmed by a propane heater with its umbilical line piercing the thick brick walls to fuel tanks beside the house, was open. An archway opened onto the sun porch, where, among the houseplants, flats of cabbage, tomato, marigold, and other seedlings greened the brown earth.

The house's inside partitions were removable wooden panels. When Beilers took their annual turn for church, the downstairs became one large room. The hand-loomed rag rugs were removed from the parlor floor, furniture pushed against the wall or moved to the porch, and benches carried in from the community's gray "bank wagon."

I admired the Amish and respected their independence and perseverance. By being willing to deliver babies at home, I felt a part of the struggle to maintain their lifestyle.

At Priscilla's bedside, I laid out a box of gloves and a sterile pack containing two clamps and a scissors, usually all the instruments needed. A disposable syringe contained the always ready Pitocin for post-delivery emergencies. An enamel washbasin to catch the placenta sat on the bureau beside a pile of baby clothes.

"We might as well sit in the kitchen," Priscilla said, buttoning a blue home-sewn housecoat over a cutoff tattered nightgown saved for her delivery. When she slipped bare feet into blue felt slippers I noticed several varicose veins. I wondered what her legs might be like 10 years from now, at age 38 and perhaps five or six children later.

"I was glad Dan gave me these slippers for Christmas," she said, stuffing loose yellow hair under a white kerchief. She drew it tight around the hair knot behind her head. Amish girls and women never cut their hair, and women cover their heads day and night according to the biblical passage in I Corinthians 11:5-15.

Priscilla selected a handful of infant clothes and blankets. She stepped around Sadie, a toddler about two years old, playing on the shining linoleum amid rag dolls dressed in Amish clothing, pot lids, and hand-painted farm animals.

"You won't be the baby much longer," Priscilla said sadly, sliding rimless glasses over her heavy nose to eyes the blue of Delft plates. She stopped to pant a moment before raising a six-pronged clothes rack from the wall behind the stove. She hung the clothes near the heat and turned two rectangular white muslin bags on top of the stove.

When I inspected the heated bags, they were soft. The contents rolled like small pebbles, but they were not as heavy. "These bags smell like corn. What are they for?" I asked feeling for kernels.

"They're corn bags. Better than hot water bottles. My feet always get cold when I'm in labor. They'll feel good later," Priscilla said.

"We might as well sit and wait," Dan said, moving into the rolling desk chair at the head of the table. He probably had been reading aloud from the open German Bible before I arrived.

Amish church meets only every two weeks, but even if it had been their Sunday to gather, the family would not have attended with Mom so near term. They were expected, however, to dress in their best clothes, read the Bible, and also keep the Lord's Day on non-church Sundays.

"We'll bring a good rocker from the parlor," Priscilla insisted.

I had refused the couch and recliner chair at the living room end of the kitchen. Instead I sat near a boy silently hunting pieces of a jigsaw puzzles at the table. Shortened to accommodate the Beiler family, I had seen these harvest tables extended to seat 20 people and covered with platters of roast beef, fried chicken, cloud-like dishes of mashed potatoes, gravy, and many vegetable and desserts.

"Emmanuel, you'll soon have that puzzle finished," Dan said.

The boy said nothing. He smiled a shy appreciative grin and placed another piece along an edge. The puzzle was on plywood so Mom could move it undisturbed at mealtime.

"Have you done any plowing?" I asked Dan.

"Had a good week of it in February; then the ground

froze again and we had the blizzard. We were pretty edgy about Priscilla. We thought of hauling her out to sister Rebecca's along the Lincoln Highway."

We talked about his 28 milk cows and 10 heifers. After the baby delivered he hoped to get to New Holland Sales Barn to buy another team of mules. Dan's lean face lit with satisfaction as he told of good tobacco prices last December.

Tobacco-selling was uncertain business. Buyers traveled the country roads hunting unsold crops. Prices fluctuated daily. After stripping, farmers loaded bales onto wagons or trucks and delivered them to the tobacco companies. Tobacco was the cash crop on many farms, but it involved nine months of work.

"I steamed and seeded my tobacco beds last fall. Most men wait 'til spring, but I like an early start. I should have plenty of plants this year. Some to sell." Dan motioned toward long muslin-covered rows in the garden outside the kitchen, bare of snow in places.

"I hope it thaws soon," Priscilla said. "I planted early cutting lettuce and radishes under the upper end of the tobacco muslin. They'll taste good in several weeks. Some say peas should be in by Saint Patrick's Day, not that I believe in it." She smiled, knowing that a sister, friend, or her mother would plant the Beilers' early seeds this year.

Priscilla brought a jar of last summer's grape juice from the cellar. I relaxed, knowing my car phone would blow the horn if I were needed.

Dan smoked a cigar, blowing billows of smoke about his chiseled lean face, tanned from hours outdoors. At 30, small lines formed beside his eyes when he laughed or squinted into the sunsplashed snow. The lines softened when he spoke to his family, but his deep voice maintained the authoritative tone defining him as head of the household.

Priscilla occupied herself with small chores. She dried the dishes and put them away, added coal to the stove and set the draft, turned the warming baby clothes. She paused to turn away from the children and pant during contractions.

Sadie became irritable. Priscilla held and amused her until nothing satisfied the child. The mother filled a bottle with milk from the propane refrigerator. She laid Sadie across her lap, sticking the diaper pins into her hair bun while changing the baby. "Makes the pins slide through the diaper easier," she said, laying Sadie in her crib beside the parents' bed.

"Is Emmanuel always this quiet?" I asked.

His black eyes watched our activities, but he had not spoken a word. The round child-face showed little emotion except concern when he caught his mother at her panting.

"Hardly," Priscilla laughed. "He usually talks up a storm. Wait 'til you go home. It isn't that he doesn't understand English. This is just his first year for it."

"Are you in first grade?" I asked the small version of his father. It amazed me that the Amish have no German accent. An outsider would not know that the Amish speak anything but the English of their surrounding neighbors.

The boy answered with a quick nod and dropped his eyes to the puzzle. For the first time he recognized my presence with a smile.

While I sat at the table drinking grape juice and munching fat salty pretzels, I found an occasional piece for the difficult "Ship At Sea" puzzle. My finds were only one-fourth the number Emmanuel found. When I praised him, his round face glowed but he remained silent. He watched intently every move I made, listening to everything the non-Amish stranger said.

"Come on, Cill," Dan teased, pulling a pocket watch onto a broad hand. "I have a herd of women in the barn that want to see me before long. It'll take me longer with the hired boy away on Sunday."

"Yes, we hit it good not to have him around today," Priscilla said. "He'll be at Georgetown to a sing tonight."

"Brother John's oldest is our hired boy. I'd rather have one older than 15, but they have to start sometime," Dan said. "Last year we had Priscilla's brother, but he married in the fall. Guess you'll be seeing his wife soon."

Priscilla winced and panted. "Time to go to bed. Let's go next door."

"You stay at the table," Dan ordered Emmanuel, closing the door behind us.

At 4:05 p.m., Priscilla delivered a seven-pound, four-ounce boy with no more than a grunt, without episiotomy or sutures.

Dan sat on the bed beside his wife. He held her hand or encouraged her through labor.

"Here is the father's share," I told Dan, handing him the basin of placenta.

"What can I do with that? The ground's frozen."

"Bury it in the manure pile. It soon disintegrates."

"Soon done. At least I won't be very late with the milking. Can you stay while I fetch Mother Fisher at the next farm?"

When Dan returned, Priscilla was comfortable with the corn bags warming her feet, and I was ready to leave. Sadie was awakening, the newborn was wrapped in his crib, and Emmanuel still sat at his puzzle. He had watched every move between bedroom and kitchen.

The day I stopped to check on the Daniel L. Beiler family, Priscilla sat in a large rocker lined with a heavy gray comforter. She held her new son, Reuben Fisher Beiler.

Everyone appeared well. As I put on my coat to leave, Priscilla laughed—as if about to divulge an intimate secret.

"After you left Sunday, we called Emmanuel in to see the new baby. He was surprised and asked, 'Where did the baby come from?' We told him that God brought it. He thought for several minutes and said, 'Is that who was here?'"

"Well, I've never been called God before," I chuckled.

"That's not all." Priscilla grinned. "He couldn't wait to go to school on Monday and tell about his new brother. He said God came to his house to bring the baby, and God was a woman."

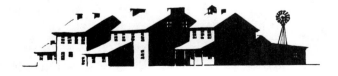

9.
Generations

Anna's new baby lay on the bed, still wet with amniotic fluid. His chubby arms and legs, flexed close to a beautiful body, waved, and kicked. But above his chin and nose, normal eyes protruded frog-like over a browless, crownless skull. He cried in high-pitched wails.

Bewildered, Levi looked at the baby and then to me. He said nothing, searching, awaiting an answer for the creature lying on the bed.

"It's a boy," I told Anna Mary flatly.

Telling the new mother her baby was not the normal, beautiful child she expected was a swallow of the bitterest medicine. This mother was a woman liked by everyone. You could not help it. Wiry, with an air of carefree happiness and generosity, Anna Mary rushed through house and garden as if work was not an effort but the pleasure for which each day was made. Curly blond hair usually escaped the edges of her white Amish cap, despite efforts to tame it into the bun at the nape of her neck. Short and slight in stature, she had brown eyes that snapped with good humor. I rarely left her house without a bag of fresh vegetables, fresh bread, or an apple snitz pie.

Anna Mary and her husband Levi R. lived in a deep hollow where Newport Road bends sharply toward Byerstown on its way to the village of Gap.

When Levi married, John S. Fisher cut 20 acres off the east end of his 90-acre farm for his oldest son. On this parcel John built a small barn, a white frame house, and two long chicken houses. Levi raised broilers for Victor Weaver's chicken plant in New Holland.

Several years in the future one of John's and Jemima's sons would take over the farm, and they would retire to the little chicken farm.

When Anna Mary sat beside my desk during her first pregnancy, we were already old friends. I had watched her grow up in the home of her parents, Barbara and Amos B. Zook, near Bard's Crossing. Her younger brothers and sisters were among the babies I delivered, and every winter flu and bronchitis seemed to plague the Zook family. I was equally familiar with John's and Jemima's family.

Anna Mary's third pregnancy was obvious at her first visit. Eighteen-month-old Barbara squirmed on her mother's lap. Johnny, age three, investigated everything in my office, particularly the holes in the electrical outlet which sent me leaping across the room to interrupt one small finger on its way to contact.

Diving over an examining table, I reached Johnny before he met the electrical charge. I set him at his mother's feet from where he scowled and threatened to cry. Barbara allowed Nurse Anna to entertain her while I confirmed what Anna Mary already knew, that she carried an active, growing baby.

"Seven months is too long to wait for a first visit," I admonished, running a finger over enlarging veins along Anna Mary's right leg. "Better get elastic stockings under these black ones. No more going barefoot for awhile."

"I rest every day when the children nap, take vitamins, and drink raspberry leaf tea. The tea makes delivery easier. I felt too good to bother a doctor."

Levi called me out to deliver their baby on a cold November night. We waited in the shadowy bedroom warmed by a propane heater. Layered blankets and baby clothes hung on chairbacks beside the kitchen stove. Barbara and Johnny slept in cribs along the wall, unaware of light or voices.

"I don't know why I'm so slow tonight. I did better with Barbara," Anna Mary complained between contractions.

Finally a head of soot-black hair bulged the perineum, and I guided a malformed baby onto the bed.

Now I knew why I had not clearly palpated the sutures on the baby's head, why Anna Mary had a longer labor.

When a baby is born at home there is no way to whisk tragedy off to the nursery and postpone reality until a stronger day. Country people steel themselves to face what is set before them.

Levi sat on the bed beside Anna Mary, watching in shocked amazement as I covered the whining baby with warm blankets and prepared to deliver the placenta. He waited for me to speak, his face rigid.

"Anna Mary," I faltered. "Anna Mary," I repeated in the gentlest tone I could find, "your baby is not normal. He has a tiny head. His head is too small." I held my breath, watching her reaction, hoping it would not endanger the last part of her delivery.

"Oh no! Let me have him. I want to see him." Tears filled her eyes as she took the baby. Gently, she pushed the blanket from his face and ran a slender finger over his black head, nearly flat, where a round skull should have been. Squinted eyes bulged where there should have been a forehead.

"What did I do to cause this? I should have come to see you earlier." Anna Mary caressed the baby's plump arms, admired his tiny fingers, kissed his cheek.

"You didn't do anything," I insisted. "You couldn't prevent this. It is inherited. You have no reason to feel guilty. Do you know of babies like this in either of your families?"

"Oh, yes," Levi said, his eyes moist. "My great-uncle Enos Kauffman had several babies like this. A cousin of Anna Mary's, Kore Esch, had one, too. Mom said they didn't live very long."

"You're right," I said. "I haven't seen any survive more than five to six months."

"You poor little thing," Anna Mary crooned sadly. Her sorrow was not for herself, but for what the baby should have become and would never be. She grieved for the short time he would be theirs, for what he might suffer, for Levi's disappointment in having and then not having another son.

The next months I saw them frequently. At first Anna Mary struggled to breast-feed little Eli, but his instinct to suckle was poor. The bottle was more successful.

"I'm not sure if he can see anymore or not," Anna Mary said at one visit. She wiggled a pacifier between his lips in an effort to comfort him. With time the baby became more irritable, cried frequently, and then began to have convulsions which required sedation. He grew except for his head, causing increased intracranial pressure.

Unfortunately I had delivered other microcephalic children among the Amish. Mary and Elias Beiler near Ronks had smallheaded boys and girls, frequent miscarriages, and three apparently normal children out of 16 pregnancies. Other families were not too different.

Achondroplastic dwarfs also were not rare. Their characteristically stubby arms and legs, and their extra fingers and toes which can be surgically removed, are not life-threatening. The usual cleft palate and lip can be corrected as well. The common occurrence of serious heat lesions, incompatible with life beyond a few weeks or years, causes the demise of most of these children. Dwarfism is frequently repeated within a family.

Joseph and Fannie Riehl had several Down's children. When the normal children grew up, they occupied their four siblings with handicaps with useful odd jobs on the farms. They were kept at home, busy, happy, and always anxious to grunt and gesture welcoming greetings to visitors.

The genetics department of Johns Hopkins University has found the Amish, with their closed society and accurate family records, to make excellent genetic studies. The University has helped the Amish community by establishing a system of reporting and recording congenital problems.

On an evening in early April, Levi telephoned from the phone booth at the end of his lane. "Can you come out? I guess the baby won't last much longer," he said.

I drove slowly through spring's humid darkness. Newly plowed fields exuded the odor of fresh earth. In wooded areas the aroma of moldering leaves hung undigested in the air. The soft thaw of day changed into night's crunching frost on the Fisher lane.

By the light of a Coleman lantern hung above the kitchen table, I saw Levi seated in his swivel chair. He rose to meet me at the sun porch door when he heard the crunch of tires on gravel.

"Come in," he said in a near whisper. His gentle face was sad and drawn, brown eyes dull and pensive. His stockinged feet made no sound on the bare linoleum. He was dressed in clean, ironed, everyday pants and shirt. After a quick smile he returned to the open Bible.

I walked through the tidy kitchen to Anna Mary, patting and rocking Eli beside the stove. When I approached she smiled faintly in recognition and laid him across her knees. As she gently unwrapped the new, fuzzy blanket, the sweet odor of fresh baby powder rose to meet me. I lifted his green dress and clean undershirt to press my stethoscope on his chest. Breath sounds were labored, rattling, and spasmodic. His skin was cool and ashen blue. Protruding more than ever, his closed eyelids did not flutter.

"He has been bad all day but slipping since supper," Anna Mary said. Her face was pale and tired but not tense. She rewrapped the baby and pressed him to her chest, the long vigil nearly finished. "I have been holding him against my shoulder since the noon meal. He seems to breathe easier that way."

Levi's mother moved ponderously but quickly around the kitchen. She pulled down the green window shades against the invading dark, undressed the other children, and put them to bed. The few words were whispered. The children obeyed Jemima silently.

John Fisher sat in a parlor rocker pulled to a darker corner of the kitchen. He rocked quietly, waiting. Occasionally he spoke to his wife in hushed words of Pennsylvania Dutch.

"My parents are on their way." Anna Mary was calm. She looked lovingly at her dying son. "At least we had him for a little while to love and care for. God is good."

The steady rocking of chairs, the ticking mantel clock, and baby Eli's labored breathing marked time in the somber room until a horse and carriage grated stones on the driveway.

Minutes later, Barbara Zook entered the room through the kettlehouse. Dressed totally in Sunday black, she moved slowly around the kitchen. Walking to Jemima seated near the table, she shook her hand. "Jemima." John rose to shake hands, "John. Levi," she spoke to her son-in-law, clasping his hand before he left to help Amos unhitch his horse and put him in the barn.

Barbara greeted me in the same way. Filled with emotion I would have preferred to hug her buxom body close and shed a tear, for we were old friends. There were no tears in that room.

To her daughter she merely spoke, "Anna Mary," in a quiet tone, but in Barbara's eyes was a depth of sympathy and understanding that needed no words. Gently, she rested a hand on Anna Mary's shoulder a moment before feeling for the large blanket pin holding her fringed black shawl closed at the neck. Carrying her stiff-boarded bonnet and the shawl into the parlor she returned with a rocking chair and sat to share the vigil.

Amos joined the group. He reverently repeated the greeting and handshaking. To his daughter he said, "How are you?" and silently took a chair beside John.

Again, rocking and ticking moved evening toward night.

I sat on the kitchen couch and waited. I didn't wait long. The baby's erratic breathing against his mother's shoulder became less frequent until it stopped. No one moved, awaiting one more breath.

The grandparents left their chairs. With Levi, they watched me examine the lifeless form on Anna Mary's lap. There were no breath sounds, but the heart continued to beat strongly for several minutes before hesitating into complete silence. When the chest became noiseless, I folded the blanket gently over the baby's body and nodded to those who shared the watch.

"A blessing he could go."

"Now he will finally have peace."

"He is in a better place. God was good to us."

"Thank you for not doing anything to give him pain or make him last longer," Grandfather Fisher said in a subdued voice.

As I closed the kitchen door softly behind me, Anna Mary still sat with her baby across her knees. Levi sat beside her.

I would call Al Furman, the funeral director, from my phone at home. The family would have another hour with their baby before the world of reality intruded on them. Tomorrow or the next day, family and neighbors would gather around a small grave.

With sadness, I felt that this would not be the last such infant Anna Mary would rock on her shoulder.

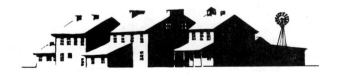

10.
The Welsh Mountains

Bugs and crawly things do not send me into spastic dances. I do not scream if a bee buzzes close or a spider drops onto my arm from the apple tree. But wrens in the grape arbor or robins nesting in the pear tree relish worms and caterpillars more than I do.

One May Sunday, I sat in church watching a fly circle and land, circle and land, on Paul Weber's bald head two pews in front. A bumblebee flew in through the half-open window and out again.

During the Epistle reading an usher handed me a message from the answering service. Nancy White in the Welsh Mountains needed me for a birthing.

The Welsh Mountains are high green hills beginning several miles below New Holland and extending eastward toward Coatesville, an hour's ride away. The hills were named for Welsh settlers who migrated into the area during the eighteenth century under a William Penn Land Grant. The people came as farmers and later owned or

worked furnaces, extracting iron from the hills. They man-
ufactured Revolutionary War cannons and ball and cast-
iron plates for Franklin stoves.

I visited and knew the mountains. Their rocky slopes of
second- and third-growth trees shaded a variety of African-
American, Puerto Rican, and white people. The names
Buzzard and Millisock, Boots and Spotts seemed as old as
the mountains themselves.

From the unfertile hills one could look out over broad
valleys of small fields, tilled mostly by Amish and
Mennonite farmers. Mountain real estate in the 1960s
could still be purchased for 10 to 15 dollars per acre. Few
noted the expansive views or the summer coolness.

At night, people living in the valleys never ventured off
State Road 897 as they drove the ridge from Blue Ball to the
crossroad village of Springville on the south. Women rarely
drove the mountain alone. Old legends were heavy with
moonshine and hidden stills, wild parties, and bloodshed.

I knew many of the hill people by name and was not
afraid, reasoning that my black bag was a passport.
Necessity made me their friend.

On that May Sunday, I left New Holland and drove four
miles across the broad farmed valley, past the airport and
Ranck's Church through Greenbank where the twisting
narrow road rises rapidly into the mountain.

At the mountain top, the road crossed Route 897 at the
old signboards. Here, a tumbledown block and wooden
house reminded me of a black woman known to many
New Holland men. After working her trade for several
decades, Flossie had moved on.

Before Public Assistance Laws were passed in
Pennsylvania, most Welsh Mountain babies were by neces-

sity born at home and by the doctor's charity. Women searched for physicians willing to deliver for lower fees or for nothing. "Pay ya on Friday" was the classic phrase. They never said which Friday, but we knew.

I drove onto 897, passing many huts in various states of propped-up and tumbledown. This morning no one came with cans or buckets to the water trough. Water fell from an old iron pipe laid to a spring farther back in the hillside. It splashed into a cement trough, overflowed into the roadside ditch and down to the valley. This spring was the only water source for most mountain people. New Holland residents frequently came with jugs to get fresh spring water.

Beyond the watering trough, I stopped my car on hardpacked earth before a shingled green cabin. Three rickety steps took me to an unstable wooden porch, weak from weather and longevity. A soap-ringed washtub sat on a wooden bench along the house wall. Three sun-bleached rockers staggered along the porch.

Remembering that I had never delivered Nancy before and concentrating on stepping around weak spots on the porch floor, I was startled by a heavy woman's voice.

"Hiya, docta. I'm Nancy's sister Annie from Coatesville. Come up ta hep out taday," a pleasant voice spoke from behind the sagging screen door. "Come in. Anythin' ya need, holla."

Annie was a rotund, matronly black woman, neatly dressed in a starched white apron and clean blue gingham dress. Her generous bosom stretched its top buttons to their limit. She had bound her hair into a tight knot behind her head.

"Come in," she repeated, smiling a grin that showed several absent teeth and brown snags of others. She held the screen door for me. It creaked a relieved sigh before slamming softly behind us.

When I stepped into the dark kitchen, a thin black boy of about 12 and a slender meager-toothed black man, drinking coffee and eating doughnuts, rose from the table. Silently, they walked into the yard and down the road.

Annie had put a teakettle to boil on the cookstove. It whistled quietly to a bucket of clothes set to boil for Monday's washing. A wide board nailed along the wall served as counter space. The distinct odor of kerosene came from a three-burner stove near the door.

As I crossed the patched and repatched linoleum floor of several undistinguishable patterns, Nancy called from one of the two bedrooms that divided the rear of the cabin.

"I'm in here, docta. Sorry ta bodder ya on Sunday," she said.

I parted stringy curtains and walked bare boards to a bed along the wall. She lay deep in the bed with little more than the curve of her pregnant abdomen, heaving breasts, and her pillowed head rising above the edges of the mattress.

My patient wore a faded red cotton dress with large white daisies tucked beneath her breasts. A flimsy sheet, gray and thin from many boilings and washings, lay across her thighs. Her face was wet with perspiration and her hair, unconfined against the pillow, stood out in several directions.

I liked Nancy. She was pleasant with a smile for any subject. Nancy worked hard to support five children by doing day work in New Holland households where, I was told, she was in great demand, as well as respected for her honesty and diligence.

"Hello, Nancy. How is it going?" I asked, dodging a light

bulb hanging in the middle of the room from a twisted cord. I took her outstretched hand and held it while her face knotted. She huffed and grunted before relaxing. Her face seemed more contorted because of a scar bridging her nose and right cheek to the jaw's curve.

"Got into a fight wid ma brudder wen ah was 12," she laughed when I had taken her history several months earlier. "Had 42 stitches from dat bottle. Jes look at me." She had rubbed a hand over the raised wide gash. "It makes ma eye water iffin ah gets cold er excited." Today she dabbed the eye with a red bandana handkerchief after each contraction.

"Annie, please bring newspapers, some plastic, and clean rags," I called.

On the dresser I found four large safety pins, and I made a pad to keep Nancy's bed clean and dry.

The oak dresser must have been more than secondhand. It stood on three legs, the fourth replaced by a chunk of stove wood. Drawer knobs were intermittent; one drawer was gone. A variety of used baby clothes covered its scarred surface.

"Tom Porter sure lit outa here wen he seen ya comin," Nancy grinned. "He's da fadder dis time. Las time, too. No use gettin married. Treats me as if we was married, anyway."

"Could you bring a chair?" I called toward the kitchen.

With a face creased by grins, Annie hustled into the room carrying a chipped veneer chair, once a fine accompaniment to a fancy dining room. She dusted its stained seat with her apron as she walked.

"Anythin else ya need?" Annie asked, trying to determine our progress.

"Nothing but this baby," I answered, laying out my packs of sterile instruments on the chair.

Nancy squeezed, puffed, and groaned. The strong scent of violets rose from her bed. It mingled with the odors of amniotic fluid, perspiration, and whiffs of kerosene wafting in from the kitchen. I wondered if she had bathed in toilet water or poured it over her pillow, and I was touched by her effort to make the sweated labor bed acceptable on a warm day.

While my patient labored, I paced between two half-open windows. Through them the dank woods smells mixed with those in the room. Between the smudged glass and grimy windowsill, I could see behind the cabin a worn path to an outhouse at the edge of the trees. The trail wound around the carcasses of several burned-out and rusted cars. Spring's green blades grew through the brown remnants of last year's grasses and the charred hulls.

It was the business of many hill folk to douse a car with kerosene, burn it out to the bare metal, and sell it for junk. From the valley it was usual to see thick black smoke rise in heavy billows and surmise that someone was burning out a car.

From the side window a patch of half-worked, cloddy earth appeared partially planted. A rusted cultivator sat where last used, and sprouts of peas, corn, and straggly beans struggled through the forest soil.

I returned to Nancy from a window tour and looked with shocked horror at the floor near my bag. As if by signal, a multitude of crawling things milled around the bare boards. Black bugs moved in from the kitchen, and a variety of winged creatures dashed about under the dresser as if I were the intruder. Along the outside wall, where it seemed the floor had ages ago separated from the house, innumerable crawling critters—slim, fat, fast, or creeping—slithered or jumped around the room.

My fascination riveted on a pure white specimen, thin and fairy-winged. It scurried around the broken dresser leg several times before heading into the room. An albino bug was a new find.

My bag!

How many varmints had already invaded its dark interior? How many nested among pill bottles, packets, and stethoscope? I snatched the bag from the floor and put it on the dresser between a pile of flannel belly bands and stacked diapers. Stretching the top, I searched the contents but saw nothing move.

My right shoulder itched. I slapped at nothing on my left leg, scratched my head.

"It's comin docta," Nancy shouted. "Come quick." She inhaled a deep breath and held it. Her face became an over-inflated balloon. Neck veins stood out like thick pencils. Her eyes bulged. Only the scar remained unchanged. Tears seeped from the eye and ran across her cheek and onto the damp pillow.

A kinky-haired, howling baby boy tumbled headfirst onto the bed and began flailing its arms and legs.

"It's here! It's all ova!" Nancy shouted above the baby's screams.

"Nancy, he's beautiful," I said. "You sure could give many women a lesson on how to have a baby."

She laughed at the compliment. Together we admired her new son. For me, an easy birth meant getting home sooner.

"Come dress him, Annie," I called.

She waited in the kitchen, anxious for this opportunity and fearful that I would omit the belly band, still in common use in the '50s. Also, she wanted the privilege of dressing her new nephew the first time.

"Be shur ta fix him in da blue outfit," Nancy insisted. "Der's a new blue blanket Missus Styer give me case it's a boy."

As I walked back across the dirt yard to my car, I remembered the host of uninvited witnesses to the birthing party.

What should I do? Suppose I took several of them home with me. They would certainly be egg-laden females. How many eggs would each female carry? How many hid in my bag, on me? I visualized a neatly itemized exterminator's bill for our large house.

During the trip back to New Holland, I found that the sights and odors of spring no longer held their usual magic. I tried to think of a plan. Only one seemed plausible.

When I did not enter the house through the garage as usual, my husband came to the open back porch to see what detained me.

A strong breeze blew from the west. I removed everything from the black bag and laid each item along the low porch wall to catch the air. I unwrapped each cloth and towel, destroyed the sterility of every pack, shook the bag, and searched its corners.

I became daring. Looking in every direction repeatedly, I stripped to the skin.

From the doorway, Pete enjoyed the performance. "Here come the neighbors home from church," he taunted. "Oh, hello, Mrs. Martin." He nodded toward the street. "Did you see that man look when he passed? Nearly had an accident," he laughed. "Jake and Mabel are coming across the lawn. They must have seen you."

I ran through the doorway and into the shower.

Years later, when newspaper headlines carried stories of daring nude dashes across campuses and through streets, I shrugged and claimed the title of New Holland's First Streaker.

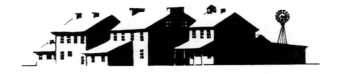

11.
Amish?

"**E**xcuse me, Mrs. Are you Amish?"

A sharp tap on my shoulder interrupted the drugstore list rotating in my head. I stood on the curb outside Rubinson's Department Store in New Holland, waiting for the street light to turn green.

"What was that?" I asked, startled from my reverie.

"Are you Amish?" repeated a bulgy, middle-aged man in blue plaid shorts.

"Who? Me?" I looked around me to be sure that I was the object of his question. The green alligator on his shirt pocket seemed to wink behind the edge of a wide camera strap.

"We thought you might be Amish. We heard that Amish come to New Holland to shop," his companion in red slacks and white halter explained.

They scrutinized me thoroughly. Their find would not go unanalyzed. I felt uneasy. Temptation raised its head. I beat it down.

The traffic light changed. To my left a woman in black bonnet and fringed shawl smothered a smile. She turned her face the other way and hurried across the street. Her dark dress lapped black lisle stockings when she stepped onto the opposite curb at Stauffer's Drugstore and disappeared into its fluorescent innards.

"No, sorry to disappoint you," I answered Mrs. Tourist. "Do I look unusual to you?"

Instead of a reply she shifted a weighty pocketbook to the other arm and pulled her hairy-legged husband down the street in search of that yet undiscovered creature, an Amish person.

Enterprising business people had made Lancaster County one of the top tourist attractions in the nation. The Amish folk with their unusual dress, horse-drawn wagons, and neat farms were the core of their ventures.

At supper I complained about it to my husband. "I could scarcely get my country calls made today. Cars and buses full of people poked along every back road." I told him about my morning experience near the drugstore. "Tourists are a nuisance, except when I am one," I said, remembering how I had ogled the Indians on western reservations and men in ten-gallon hats as they walked the streets of small Arizona towns.

"Tourists will be tourists," Peter said, reaching for another drumstick.

"Lydia Ebersole told me a good story in the office today," I continued. "Last week she and two of her children were driving home from the town of Intercourse in the market wagon. Near Applebutter Hill, a car with New York license plates passed her, then pulled in front of her horse, and stopped on the road. A woman in shorts jumped out, pushed a camera nearly into the buggy, and snapped a picture. The horse shied, jumped, and swung that carriage against the open car door. It bent the door hinge and scraped some paint off the car. It split a front corner off the market wagon, too."

"Could Lydia get home okay? It's a wonder the horse didn't run away with them."

"That's not the worst," I said. "A big man with a Brooklyn accent sprang from behind the wheel and shouted, 'What's da matta wid ya? Can't ya keep da hoss where he belongs? Look what ya did ta my new Cadillac. I hope ya got insurance. Ruthie, get 'er name and phone number.'"

I laughed. "You should hear Lydia tell the story."

Glossy buses slid over narrow country roads. Their passengers clicked cameras at trim-rowed cemeteries, covered bridges, and gray carriages of Amish who hid their faces. The hordes of invaders emptied wallets at roadside stands full of fresh jams and vegetables scarcely parted from the vine. They brought Amish souvenirs imprinted "Made in Taiwan" and gorged themselves in all-you-can-eat "Amish" restaurants.

Every tourist seemed to send two friends on the next bus. They shed cash like an oak drops fall leaves. Bus loads from Baltimore and Philadelphia hunted country markets for whoopie pies, dried corn, sweet balogna, and shoo-fly pies.

Europe, Asia, Long Island, Boston. People came to spend lazy summers in motels and campgrounds. Some formed friendships with Amish families. On hot August days they helped in dusty hayfields or speared tobacco. They shared hearty meals at bountiful tables, turned frosty tubs of ice cream, or chauffeured buggydriving friends to town on errands.

"Amish are people like the rest of us," I said, rising to clear the table. "We all share the same pleasures and disappointments. If only outsiders didn't treat them like freaks."

Abram Miller called from the phone booth beside his smithy. "Daughter Miriam's here visiting. Her boy Abner has a fever and sore throat. How soon can you come out?"

Abe and Fannie reared 11 children at his home place. Like his father, he worked a blacksmith shop on a pie-shaped piece of land large enough for the smithy, a small white barn, and a gray shingled house. There was also space for a generous garden and pasture for Bud, the sorrel driving horse, and Dottie, the Holstein cow.

Frequently I took out-of-town guests to watch Abe shoe fidgety horses or mend wobbly wagon wheels. By instinct he seemed to protect his magnificent white beard from the forge's flying sparks.

Big Abe he was called. He was thick limbed, heavy bodied, powerful. His voice rang loud and clear as the old bell in the nearby Zeltenreich Church tower.

By necessity Abe had learned to deal with tourists. At one time strangers were welcome in his shop. Later he hung an irregularly lettered sign above the long, sliding doors: NO TOURISTS ALLOWED.

Tourists had swarmed thoughtlessly over everything in the smithy. They filled pockets with costly nails or anything that fit pocket and purse. The privilege to watch hot metal bend under Abe's tapping hammer, hear a red-hot horseshoe sizzle in the tub of murky water when it tempered, or see the shoe fitted and hammered onto a newly pared hoof was denied visitors.

When afternoon office hours were finished, I drove

through the August afternoon toward Zeltenreich cross-road south of New Holland.

Behind Abe's wedge of property a spiny ridge arose from the earth which continued eastward and became the Welsh Mountains. A stony hill of rocks and bushes hung like a speckled curtain over the north edge of his pasture, where Mill Creek in its infancy emerged between banks of granite limestone and grayflecked quartz. Thicket coverings of sumac, blackberry, and elderberry hid patches of earth.

From this humid wilderness, Mill Creek staggered onto a broad valley of patchwork fields. Random barns with tall silos sat with brick or stone farmhouses.

The creek turned and returned through Abe's pasture. At the dam it turned the undershot wheel which pulled a long wire attached to a pump at the well. Without electricity, water was pumped in spurts into a tank on the ridge, then ran by gravity into the buildings below.

Past the dam, water lingered in lazy puddles under the old bridge which rattled under every carriage and thundered at cars and trucks.

The clatter of the plank floor restored my maundering mind. Abe's house sat beyond the bridge. It rose like a gray rock from the manicured lawn, cropped close to its roots by Fannie's hand-pushed reel mower. Beds of petunias, geraniums, asters, and coleus in boisterous colors edged the house and yard.

I parked beside the smithy and the pile of chunky coal for the forge. It was the last space amid a profusion of carriages, buggies, and wagons.

The yard between house and barn was a Grandma Moses painting come to life. I skirted a group of barefoot boys pitching horseshoes in the gravel drive and wondered how many toes would go to bed bandaged after this contest of flying iron.

In the shade of the barn, tables of varied heights and sizes sat on the grass. Several young girls covered them with plaid or striped tablecloths in red, green, and yellow.

Fannie stood on the walk, arms akimbo. She directed a flow of daughters, daughters-in-law, and granddaughters in Pennsylvania Dutch, as they streamed in and out of the kitchen carrying trays of pickled red beet eggs, bacon-dappled potato salad, quivering jellos, amber applesauce, fresh peaches, chocolate cakes, pies of cherry and apple.

I picked my way through a maze of croquet wickets that three adolescent girls had pushed into the turf. We exchanged hellos. Two little girls in blue dresses, whom I recognized as Abe's Isaac's children, ran to Fannie shouting, "Mommy, Mommy, Dr. Frau ist day."

I saw no feet with shoes, nor did I hear English spoken until Fannie noticed me and switched speech. "Hello, Doctor. Come in. Abner is in the *schtubb*." She continued her work. "Sadie, bring out the bread. Salome, we need knives and forks. Annie, where'd baby Joel go?"

Beyond the gray-haired Fannie, Miriam met me and led the way to her sick son in the parlor. It was the only cool, quiet room in the house.

"The poor boy just lies on this couch all day. He's hot too," Miriam said. She tossed loose cap strings over the back of a blue dress. Her brown eyes widened in the dim room.

"How long has he been sick?" I asked, lifting a dripping washcloth from Abner's forehead.

"He complained of some sore throat last week. He's

worse today. We hated to stay home and miss the family picnic; 62 of us here today. Mom insisted we call you." She smiled and pushed a strand of black hair under her white cap.

Abner whimpered as I palpated swollen glands. *"Maul uff,"* I said, looking at large white-spotted tonsils. *"Dreh rum."*

"Mam," Abner whimpered. His child face pleaded, but he reluctantly obeyed. Miriam held the four-year-old's hand while I pushed a plunger of penicillin into his buttock.

"Give him these pills as it says on the package."

"Canst du Deitsch schwetza?" Miriam asked. She helped Abner tuck his shirttail and button his broadfalls.

"No." I laughed. *"'Essa'* and *'gelt'* are all the words I need to know. But you can't buy or sell me."

Miriam offered me a moisture-beaded glass of cold peppermint tea when we walked through the kitchen. Peppermint grew in farm meadows or gardens and was the summer drink of most farm families. Its pungent aroma blended with the spicy odor of baked beans in the oven. My stomach rolled with hunger, and I wished I could join this gathering.

At an outside cellar door three half-grown boys struggled with a two-gallon ice cream churn. Frost covered the can; salt water spilled down the steps. Now I was sure I wanted to be a Miller for the day.

"Sure glad you could get out to see Abner," Fannie said when I passed her in the yard. "How 'bout stayin' to supper?"

"Mighty tempting but you have enough people. Look at all these hungry men sitting here."

I knew all of Big Abe's sons and sons-in-law. They sat in a cluster of bearded men under an elm tree on benches and chairs or in the grass. They talked, watched the women set out food, and kept the toddlers out of mischief. "Hey Doc, grab a plate," several called out.

Desire mingled with the odor of hamburgers on a grill. The grumbling in my stomach persisted. "Looks good but I don't think you have enough," I laughed.

A car full of strangers interrupted our jesting. A Buick with a Massachusetts license plate slowed on the berm of the road and stopped beside the yard. Big Abe left the smoking hamburgers and strolled barefooted across the grass. His huge frame towered above the automobile as he asked their business. Abe's long beard fluttered in the afternoon air.

"Can I help you? Where do you want to go?" he asked.

"We want to see some Amish people. Can you tell us where to find them?"

The old patriarch stood erect, pushed a thumb under a suspender and furrowed his brow. He looked left toward the bridge then right toward the crossroad. Thoughtfully he stroked his beard. Sweeping a massive arm across his chest he pointed, voice clear and emphatic, "If you take that road south you'll come to the town of Intercourse. I think you'll find some over there."

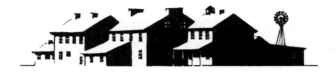

12.
Hopeless

For the first time in my career, I had to give up and concede to a hopeless situation.

I felt foolish, embarrassed, and frustrated, perched a lofty four feet above road level at one-thirty in the morning. Embarrassed because I had never had an accident or faced a problem I could not conquer. Frustrated because Edna and Henry Horst, a Mennonite family two miles farther down Log Cabin Drive, expected me.

"Better come right away. Edna woke up in labor and is moving fast," Henry said when he called from a neighbor's telephone.

"How's your road?" I asked. A January blizzard three days before had closed all thoroughfares. Some back roads were still impassable.

"Come in from Route 322," he answered. "Come soon."

Henry's warning and Edna's baby number five left no time to linger in a warm bed. I slid from under the warm covers trying not to disturb my sleeping husband. Every

bedtime I laid out clothing for the next day or the night-
time interruptions. The wool dress lying on a rocking chair
slid cold over warm skin, and I shivered.

Folded in the back of a bureau drawer, I still keep a pair
of tights I wore on frosty winter trips. They were a special
order from Sears Roebuck when leotards were not in
vogue. The insulated waffle-textured pantyhose came only
in bright red and rarely matched anything else I wore.
Warmth meant more than appearance when the thermometer outside our bedroom window read minus two
degrees.

When I went down the hall, I stopped to check baby
Paul, fourth of the Kaiser tribe. A brassy cough, probably
due to hours on his sled, had concerned me at bedtime. I
brushed a finger over his windburned cheeks and tucked
blankets around his shoulders.

Pulling on boots, heavy coat, and gloves, I headed out of
town on North Railroad Avenue. Roadbanks were piled
high with snow where plows had worked around the clock
to open clogged highways. On main roads, surfaces were
clear. Snow had melted or worn away. In spots, the day's
thaw refroze into patches slippery as greased glass.

The sky was clear, and a full moon reflected on white
fields so brilliantly that headlights were unnecessary. Dark
houses intruded on the white countryside. Skaters had
gone home from Sensenig's Mill Pond, but their paths of
shoveled snow left geometric designs along wiggly cleared
ice trails.

Past the mill, I turned onto Log Cabin Drive. The road
was dry. Only one car could drive between the snowbanks.
At intervals, wider areas had been cleared to allow cars to
pass.

For an eighth of a mile, the road cut through white fields, turned toward a farm beside the stream, then made a sharp bend and followed the Conestoga Creek. Silent summer cabins squatted in a fringe of trees like pheasants hunched in a summer grass field.

Beneath the trees, the sun had not penetrated shadows long enough to melt the snow left by plows. Trucks and cars had packed it into a slick sheet. Near the curve I unexpectedly met this glassed snow, slippery as ice. It shone suddenly in the headlights, glistening on the snow-canyon's floor.

The car seemed to pick up speed as it catapulted toward the curve. Braking would have hurled me into a snowbank. For a moment I felt airborne, then settled with a crunch on the piled snow at the road's edge. It was useless, but I started the stalled engine and gunned it into reverse. Only snow moved under the rear wheels.

Unbelieving, I sat a moment. Now what? How could I reach the Horst home? It was cold along the creek, and, by the moonlight filtering through spectral trees, I could see packed snow shining on the road ahead. I doubted if I could stand; I certainly could not walk any distance. Even if I could reach the nearby farmhouse, it would take considerable time to arouse the sleeping householder, wait for him to dress and hitch a horse, and then drive the several miles of slippery creekside road. It looked impossible to reach Edna in time.

I imagined Henry, short and portly, pacing stocking-footed across the Horst's kitchen linoleum. Occasionally he would stop to melt a patch of frost from a window with a flattened hand and peer into the quiet night, hoping to see headlights. "Relax, hold back," he would call to Edna in the adjoining bedroom.

Edna would be more calm than her nervous husband who was always jittery when his wife had a baby. At these times I had seen Henry forget where the simplest items were kept—a wash basin, a bar of soap or towels. He usually sputtered around underfoot, cast shadows on my work, held the lantern at the wrong places, or totally disappeared when I needed him most.

There seemed only one solution to my snowbound dilemma. Resigned that I could not get to Horsts, I picked up the car phone beside me and called Dr. John Martin. He conducted a general practice in Blue Ball. We covered each other on days off, emergencies, and vacations. This was an emergency.

"John, it's a dirty trick on a cold night, but I'm stuck on a snowbank. Could you deliver Edna Horst for me?"

Silence, a grunt, a smothered laugh, and an audible chuckle.

Swallowing failure went down like a dose of castor oil. I gave him directions and hoped he could beat the baby.

Next I called home. On the third ring a sleepy voice answered, "Hello. Dr. Kaiser's office."

"Pete, I'm stuck on a snowbank. Can you come get me?"

"Ugh. Sometime before breakfast," he answered, only half amused.

The phone settled back in its cradle, and I remembered past years when there was no car phone and I struggled to reach a public telephone or, instead, aroused a sleeping family if a crisis arose. Doctors kept a mental list of available public phones within their areas. Many non-Amish farmers had telephones in barns or milk houses for shared use by Amish neighbors. This eliminated interruption of family life by phone users. These telephones were not publicized.

My station wagon was warm, and I was dressed for cold. I relaxed and waited rescue.

Only a car's length ahead, the creek mumbled beneath its ice lips. To the left a farm huddled dark against the snow. Upstream, I saw the shadowy outline of Sensenig's mill. Unblemished snow fields rose toward Ephrata, five miles away. Downstream, skeleton trees hovered over the road as it twisted with the Conestoga creek past the cold and vacant cottages.

Half dozing, I thought over past years of rural practice. Most memorable experiences were related to weather— high water, deep snow, ice, the seduction of balmy days. When Velma Good needed me after a December blizzard, I had borrowed Jeep and driver to travel through fields and fences cut for sleighs and wagons to haul milk to plowed highways. Mary Todd, far in the Welsh Mountains, called during a spring thaw when mud was axle deep, and to stick in her lane would have meant a neighbor's tractor or team of horses. Levi Stoltzfus sleighed me in a biting blizzard to treat his son's croup. Snow cut our scarf-wrapped faces like knives and gave new meaning to romanticized sleighs on Christmas cards.

Summer days I loitered along country roads to enjoy fresh-cut grasses drying in the sun or stopped to pick road-bank violets and honeysuckle growing like weeds. Their pungent odor contrasted fields of freshly spread manure.

On a hill east of Strasburg, I often stopped for an aerial view of farms. I photographed green-rowed cornfields, surging grainfields, herds of Holsteins. In the fall I snapped yellow piles of corn between fat shocks. From the rise, patches of plowed earth checkered green squares of winter wheat. Plodding teams pulled wagons, harvesters, and grain drills across the valley like ants. Stately farmhouses, set in stands of elms or maples, mothered white barns with silos and clustered outbuildings. Woods and meadow streams splotched the rolling countryside, changed season to season, and never tired me.

In the cooling car, I imagined the calls and clatter of spring birds, the click and whir of mowers lopping grasses, the autumn whine of cutters shooting corn into tubular silos.

A mother raccoon and five young ones walked single file down dawn's path; a pair of red foxes leaped across the road with great bushy tails streaming against the sunrise.

I smiled, remembering Bill, stooped and aged. Each spring the old black man brought me sprigs of trailing arbutus. His toothless smile meant more than the rare blossoms held in his contorted hand. The Welsh Mountains do not relinquish secrets easily.

An hour passed on the snowbank. The station wagon became cold. If the exhaust pipe were covered by snow it would be dangerous to run the engine. Where was John? Why hadn't he passed? Was he, too, stuck in the snow? Why was Pete so long in coming? Of course he had to arouse a baby sitter.

For the first time, headlights moved up the creek toward me. A red sports car stopped under my roost. John, dressed in a heavy brown wool jacket and cap, stopped and stepped into the snowbank. Standing with one boot in the car he brushed snow from a pant leg.

"Hi there. You okay?" He cocked his head and smiled, leaning across the convertible's canvas top. "Need help, a ride home?"

"No, thank you. How did things go at Horsts?"

"Fine. I walked in just in time. Henry's okay, too." John laughed and coughed a cloud of frost into the air.

"I'm grateful. I'll stop in there tomorrow. Shame to get you out of bed."

"I'll do the same for you some night." He laughed, shot more vapor, and slid behind the wheel, stomping a foot against the open door.

"Thanks." I knew he would do it.

"I drove in through Farmersville on the other side," he said. "The road's still drifted and barely open there."

As John drove away another set of headlights stopped on the highway and waited to enter Log Cabin Drive. A red van lettered Spring Gulch Campground stopped at my curve and Peter stepped out.

"Hello lady. What are you doing up there?"

"Took the wrong turn last summer," I quipped.

"That chain I brought to pull you out is useless. Call B. Z. Mellinger in the morning. He'll come out with a tow truck and winch you off." Breath hovered around his head in smoky frost. An immense tan corduroy coat seemed to direct his large body. He moved with ease along the icy road. His eyes, barely visible under a hooded wool cap, twinkled with amusement when he took my bag and helped me from the drift.

"Hated to get you out of bed," I apologized.

"I'll get even. Knew it would happen some day," he teased.

Mortified, I went home to a bed that should have been warm at that hour. Worst of all, two men had vowed revenge.

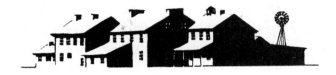

13.
Trouble in Triple

"I'm sure I'm pregnant," Ethel said. She stared at the floor, slender fingers replacing a strand of raven hair that dared stray from its place.

"We'll soon find out," I said.

The February day when I first met Ethel was clear and warm. My office schedule looked like a passenger list for the last train out of town before a predicted disaster. The sun warmed the winter-sodden earth, sending exhilarating promises of spring to its cold-weary creatures. Farmers hitched their teams to plows for a day of early tilling; women cleaned garden patches or came to town on postponed errands. People bustled about like cows released from their stanchions on the first day of spring pasture.

Ethel Madison matched the day. She carried sunshine, dignity, and poise into my consultation room like an exotic orchid on a silver tray.

"Are you unhappy about a pregnancy?" I asked, admiring her finely molded face, a perfect tawny oval.

Ethel wore no label of "Trouble Ahead" or "Danger." Patients seldom do. Perhaps it is better, they reason, to keep doctors on the alert, wary, and watching.

"I just got a promotion to private secretary," she said, pursing finely painted lips that matched the carmine fingernails she nervously tapped on my plate-glass desk. "I wanted several years of career before we started a family."

"An ambition I can understand," I said, thinking of my two-year-old playing in the sandbox beneath the old pear tree.

"I'm not as happy as my husband. Gary is glad about a baby, but he is studying for the Methodist ministry and I expected to help him finish college." She carefully dabbed tears from her eyes without smudging mascara or eye shadow. "Gary loves children."

Gary came with his wife on her next prenatal visit. He was a quiet, concerned man. His tan suit fit broad shoulders and trim body like a television advertisement for a men's store. He was handsome with curly black hair falling over a wide unfurrowed brow. Leading Ethel by an elbow he walked with firm step. He was direct and asked many questions.

"We're looking forward to this baby," he said, smiling at Ethel.

During the months of visits that followed, I learned to know Ethel and Gary well. She continued employment at New Holland Machine Company. As her pregnancy progressed, Ethel spoke less frequently of her work and more often of the coming birth, preparations for the baby's arrival, and baby showers. Her enthusiasm grew as fall approached.

In mid-September Gary brought his wife into the office, ready for the hospital. During her labor he sat holding her hand, encouraging her when she tired. In the early 1960s husbands still paced and smoked in waiting rooms while their wives delivered.

When the nurse wheeled Ethel from the delivery room, Gloria Jean lay bundled in her arms, strenuously sucking her fist. The mother appeared crisp and fresh. No one seeing Ethel's meticulously combed hair and freshly applied make-up, would have guessed she had finished 10 hours of labor.

The second day following delivery, Ethel complained of vague pains, not "feeling well." Her blood pressure elevated and she became feverish. Twelve miles from the hospital and busy in the country, I obeyed the inner voice that advised me to refer this case. I felt certain all complications would soon be reversed. Daily hospital visits kept me abreast of Ethel's condition. Her blood pressure and fever rose.

One trouble seems to invite others to keep it company. I was in the office removing a full leg cast from a patient when the door between the office and our kitchen rattled with heavy, urgent knocking. The office receptionist ran to open the door.

"I can't find baby Paul anywhere," Gertrude, our housekeeper, cried in panic. The announcement sounded through our rooms like a bullhorn. She was near tears.

I turned off the buzzing cast-cutter and ran to the door. "Did you look in the neighbors' yards?"

"Yes, and called everywhere," she wailed. "I went upstairs to vacuum the front bedroom, looked out the window, and he was gone in only five minutes." She held up five shaking fingers, then wrapped them in her gingham apron.

"He can't have gone far," I said, consoling her. "We'll look. We'll find him."

The patient and her cast could wait; she would not run away. The office receptionist and I joined the search.

The outside telephone bell clanged as I hurried over the back porch. It was a call from the hospital.

"Ethel Madison is worse today. Her temperature is higher. I wanted you to know. She's a sick woman."

"Thanks for calling," I said limply, hanging up the phone.

I rejoined the child hunt, ran to Main Street several times, looking in both directions for red overalls and a yellow jacket. I rang the brass porch bell, a "come-home" signal no Kaiser child or dog dared ignore. People on Railroad Avenue, a mile away, must have heard it. No child appeared.

Our driveway sloped toward the street. Had Paul ignored a strictly enforced family law that forbade crossing the yellow line, painted where the incline began? Why didn't Ethel respond to treatment? Where could Paul be hiding?

The crew of searchers called the child's name, knocked on doors, searched and re-searched corners, under bushes.

Mable Horst, next door, saw us hunting and came out to help, broom in one hand, dust cloth in the other. "Lookin' for Paul? I saw 'im in the sandbox. He'll come back; mine always do. Maybe he's hidin'." She threw her dust rag over the porch railing and began to lift bushes with her broom handle.

Several times I passed the waiting room windows. Patients stared, expecting me to be in the office. The news spread. A handful came out to help hunt, speculate, or sympathize. Some told "lost children" stories.

How could a child disappear so fast? Why did Ethel's condition keep going downhill? Twenty minutes seemed like hours.

The weather was damp and cold. An equinoctial storm from the northeast was predicted for tomorrow. The sky was ragged gray. The sharpening wind felt like rain any minute.

Would Ethel be improved tomorrow? Maybe she needed more time for the antibiotics to work? What had happened to Paul?

I rang another volley of bell into the neighborhood. The other three children had never wandered away. I took frustration out on the bell thong.

If our search party had been unable to find the toddler, there was only one answer. He had been kidnapped. Some thug believed the word "doctor" meant "money." It was my fault that the child disappeared. The thought struck me like a slap in the face. Kidnapped.

The first raindrops splashed on the concrete walk near the porch.

As I stopped clanging the bell and turned to telephone the New Holland police, a car climbed the driveway and parked under the pear tree. A little boy, dressed in red pants and yellow jacket, slid to the ground. He clutched a one-eyed, frazzled teddy bear by its limp neck.

"I thought you might be missing this one," Jean Sensenig, a patient living a half-mile toward town, said.

"Paul," I shouted, running to hug the lost, kidnapped child.

"I found him trudging along toward downtown," Jean said. "He was going to the ''tore.'"

The baby reached for Gertrude. He wiped her wet eyes with his fist.

"Where were you going?" she asked, smiling.

"To 'tore to buy Teddy baby food."

"But you didn't have any money. How could you buy it?" the housekeeper asked, kissing him over and over on his red cheeks.

"Oh, oh," he murmured. "Can you give me some?"

"He got into my car without hesitating," Jean said.

I thanked her profusely. In a town in which everyone had at least heard of other town members, and where we did not lock our house doors during the 30 years we lived there, it was difficult to inscribe mistrust in our children.

The next morning a wind-driven northeaster smacked against the window panes. Water seeped through the east waiting room wall, blistering the plaster behind peeling wallpaper. Its secret entrance is still an enigma. We set chairs against that wall to hide our battle with the rain.

Esla, dressed in the green uniform of a Junior Girl Scout, pranced around me as I dressed. Several times she admired her image in the bathroom mirror, turning to one side and then the other. She inspected her back with a hand mirror.

"How do I look?" our older daughter asked.

"You won't look right with crooked pigtails. Stand still."

"Is my tie straight, Mommy?"

"You look fine. I never saw a nicer Scout. Beautiful," I answered, wrapping the final rubber band around a braid. I dismissed her with a kiss on her cheek.

Sharing Elsa's happy mood was difficult. I thought of Ethel, lying in her isolation room, her fever not responding to antibiotics. Each time I called the hospital, the answer was the same, "No change," or, "Fever up a bit." My night's sleep had been spasmodic.

I feigned happiness on my daughter's great day, her television debut. The New Holland Junior Girl Scout Troop was scheduled for a Saturday interview, a five-minute appearance.

As we drove through Bareville, Leola, Leacock, and into Eden, Elsa chattered and questioned, "Will the lights be hot and bright? How long will it take? Are the cameras very big?"

Windshield wipers on the station wagon slapped the unrelenting rain, chanting "Quick-quick, Sick-sick." Reaching the hospital became the most important business of the day.

"Pick you up in an hour. Wait in the doorway, out of the rain, if you finish before I get back," I told Elsa, dropping her off at Channel 8 studios on South Queen Street.

Her green knee socks were already disappearing through the brass-trimmed doors as I pulled away and hurried across Lancaster to the hospital.

Telephone conversations had not prepared me for Ethel's room. My patient appeared much worse. She lay limp and hollow-faced, the usual luster gone from her eyes. I saw in them an abstract vacancy I had seen in dying patients. For the first time she did not greet me with a quip. Hot dry skin confirmed the temperature recorded on her chart.

Ethel managed a smile. When I walked to the bed, she clenched my hand. It was like grasping a glowing ember. She pulled me close, eyes searching, fear and panic in her voice.

"Tell me. Will I die? I can feel it. I know I will," she whispered, breathing fast through cracked lips. She held me tighter, attempting to squeeze out the truth.

With dread, I remembered a young mother during intern days. She had awakened during the night, trembling. Although every examination was normal, she was sure she was dying. The nurses had called me, and the patient begged me not to leave her. She insisted I hold her in my arms. I did, listened, consoled, and comforted her until the sedative relaxed her and she fell asleep. Two days later she died of a heart lesion for which pregnancy had not been advised.

Ethel's morbid state consumed my thoughts as I watched Gary, standing at the foot of her bed, dressed in the loose white scrub gown of the isolation room. I saw tears in his eyes when his wife spoke of death. Dark fatigue lines rimmed his brow and face between cap and mask. He understood that Ethel's premonition raced toward probability.

"You will not die," I said, hiding behind my mask and formal bedside manner.

I compared the vivacious girl of past months with this collapsed woman lying gaunt in bed, hair mussed and stringy against the pillow. Surrounded by a rigging of tubes, wires, and bottles she was another person.

I held Ethel's hand and prayed for a miracle.

Outside Room 101 I pulled off isolation clothes and dipped my hands in disinfectant solution. In the hall and at the nurses' station, silence saturated the atmosphere. A patient was critical. Gloom and helpless frustration dominated the area.

The consulting specialist on Ethel's case touched my elbow as I searched her thick chart for hope. "Notice on the laboratory sheet that her infection is also sensitive to Chloramphenicol. We have held it as the antibiotic of last choice because of its possible side effects. But now we will start it immediately by intravenous."

When I passed fellow staff members in the hall, they shot silent glances in my direction. I wondered if they meant, "What happened" or "Glad she isn't my patient."

Time. My Girl Scout. I looked at my watch. An hour and a half since I had deposited her on South Queen Street.

I did not expect to find the disheveled child who crouched in the doorway at Channel 8. Her jacket hung open and crossways on her shoulders. The hair we had carefully combed flew in wisps beneath her askew beret. Grimy hands rubbed a tear-streaked face and red swollen eyes. She shook with sobs.

"Mommy, Mommy," she wailed in jerks. "Where were you so long?" She slid onto the seat beside me. "Did you forget me?"

"Were you afraid? Is that what upset you?" Guilt, heavier than the steady rain, soaked my conscience. "Did you think I forgot you?"

"Yes! No!" she cried, snuggling into my arms. "I missed it. The television was changed to yesterday. Nobody told me." She shook with spasms.

I wiped the wet face and buttoned her coat. I could have sat holding Elsa's trembling body close for a long time, sharing our distress and tears, but traffic blowing its horns poured around the square onto North Queen Street.

Our return to New Holland was dismal. Rain in fierce gusts blew across Route 23, filling ditches and flooding meadows. When would it stop?

I tried to think of lunch, the four children and Peter to feed. Tomato soup sounded right for the day.

After the baby was bedded for a nap, a circuit of house

calls filled the afternoon. Postpartum patients expected a cheerful doctor. I felt like an actress.

This was the darkest day of my career.

Five years later, Gloria Jean, trimmed in ruffles and ribbons, skipped into my office. Her blue eyes matched the clear June day.

"I'm not sick. I don't need any shots," she boasted.

"I'll be glad to find a shot for you," I said, laughingly.

"No, it's Mommy. She wants to get a baby." Tidy combed curls bounced against her neck.

Ethel nodded, smiling, "I'll order one without any complications this time, please."

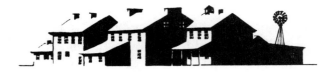

14.
Finances

The mantel clock above the kitchen table confirmed 60 minutes to feed my family before evening office hours. Enough time.

I dropped three sliced carrots, two chopped celery stalks, and a diced onion into the supper stew. They sank like stones in a mill pond.

The baby I balanced on my left arm suckled with gusto. She grinned a toothless smile and chortled happily, milk trickling across her fat chin and into the creases of her neck. I smiled and rubbed my nose against hers, wishing I could spend the whole hour in play, before five months became five years, or 15.

The grating of iron-rimmed wheels and the clop of horse hoofs on the driveway returned reality with a start. Probably a husband coming to pick up his wife, a patient from my afternoon office hours. Nearly 10 years of medical practice in rural Pennsylvania had not dulled my fascination with horses and wagons or the people who drove them.

Knocking resounded through the kitchen like the stutter of an air hammer. Quickly, I set the baby in her playpen and zippered my dress, hurrying to the door to see what life-threatening emergency interrupted my few kitchen moments.

Old Sol Zimmerman stood on the porch, his hand raised for another volley. I should have known. Sol always came at his convenience, always at the back door when I was in the house. He never went to the front door during office hours where the receptionist could attend his business.

"Good afternoon, Sol," I said, stealing a quick look at the clock. "Come in. What can I do for you?"

Sol acted as self-appointed financial manager for his 12 grown children, so I was sure he had come to pay a bill.

"Hello, Kaiser. No, I'll stay out here. This will only take a minute. I wanta pay ya for what we owe ya for Lucy, Henry's wife." He shuffled his heavy work shoes on the porch floor. By their noticeable odor and tufts of straw along the shoe edges, I knew he had spent the afternoon at the weekly cow sale in New Holland.

"Fine, Sol. But I'll have to hurry today."

No disrespect was intended by his dropping the prefix "Doctor." It was the custom of many plain people.

"How much do we owe ya?" The old man reached a scrawny hand inside his tattered coat and extracted a battered checkbook. Scratching about in an outer pocket, like a squirrel scraping fall leaves for hickory nuts, he found a pen.

I shifted impatiently from one foot to the other.

"What's the amount?" Sol moved a cud from right cheek to his left and squinted through shaggy eyebrows like a sheep dog hunting a stray ewe. He slowly sat on the wooden porch bench.

"Excuse me. I have to get your bill from the office files," I said.

On returning from the front of the house, I dropped diced potatoes into the stew. Meat and vegetables rolled in an eddy. The vapors stirred hunger pangs. My visitor was taking too much time.

"Ya sure about that?" Sol asked, looking at the sum and shaking his pen. His grubby hand poked through a frayed sleeve like a gopher from its grassy burrow. He tilted his black-brimmed hat, soiled with sweat and dust, and watched me, his thin face so glum I expected tears to seep from the sallow brown eyes.

"Yes, that is exactly right," I answered, trying to maintain a Mount Rushmore expression.

"Remember, things didn't turn out so good this time. Lucy had to go to the hospital. Hospitals cost dear. We plain folk don't have insurance like your people. Hospitals are hard on us farmers. We don't have no baby this time."

Sol and I played the game several times a year when he paid a family bill. I stepped into the kitchen and lowered the heat under the stew.

"Yes, I feel bad about the baby, but no one called me until Lucy's water dripped a week and she had a fever. Seven-month babies are a special problem when conditions are good."

"We thought it would clear up without a doctor." His stubbled face remained unsmiling and sad. "How much is the bill?"

"The same as five minutes ago. The same as the last baby. You're lucky to have Lucy home again."

Sol grunted and crossed his legs. His faded pants, patched and repatched in shades of black denim, hung loosely against his calves. He set his pen to the check. "We should'a brung that baby home and buried it in a corner of the yard like we wanted. No sense payin' an undertaker for that little thing." His pen made no mark on the paper.

"It's the law." I explained that any pregnancy over 16 weeks requires a funeral director. The hour was escaping rapidly.

My visitor took a pair of wire-rimmed glasses from a vest pocket and carefully adjusted them behind each ear before sliding them over the hump on his nose. "Things get more expensive every year." His voice became a whimper.

"Don't forget I took Lucy to the hospital in my car. That saved an ambulance fee. I brought her home again, too, so you didn't have to pay someone to go get her."

Sol pursed dry lips, stained tobacco-brown, as if tasting something sour. "Lucy and Henry have 14 young'uns. That takes a heap of money. It's good Lizzie and I live at the other end of the house. Keep an eye on things."

"I have expenses, too," I said, imitating his tone. "I pay two women in the office, a hired girl in the house, gasoline and car bills. I need several tel—"

"Yes. Yes. How much did you say?" His pen wrote across the paper.

It was after his first back porch visit, seven years previously, that I had learned about Solomon Zimmerman. When evening office hours were over I told my nurse about the pitiful man who came to the back door. I had greatly reduced his fee, feeling guilty at accepting money from a family in such obvious poverty.

"Lucy and Henry's home is one of the barest in Lancaster County," I said, remembering their home birthing. "They haven't a single luxury. Children run around everywhere.

Chickens scratch through the yard and sit on the porch. And poor Lucy is just a skinny shadow."

Elsie Good snorted. "No wonder—she's thin, overworked, and always pregnant. What did you think of Henry?"

"Why?" I heard no pity in her voice. "He seems to be awkward, sluggish, doesn't talk much. He scarcely looked at me when I spoke to him. I guess Lizzie and Sol keep a roof over their heads."

"You feel guilty taking Sol's money?" Elsie laughed. She had been born and reared east of New Holland and seemed to know everyone. "Why that old guy owns at least four farms that I know about. He never dresses in anything but tatters and shaves every two weeks for church. He wears his stubble like a badge of honor."

"And I thought he was miserably poor. He complained about the cost of everything, especially my fee. He's not indigent?"

"No, Sol keeps a tight rein on his money and his farms. Henry can't make a decision. Like the rest of their church people they speak only Pennsylvania Dutch at home. Henry rarely leaves the farm so he seldom speaks English. He works hard for Sol. You would scarcely know he finished the eighth grade."

"Does Sol give Henry any money?"

"I doubt if it's very much. Henry will get his twelfth share when Sol dies. Not before. Henry doesn't know any better."

"Whew. Is the old man honest?" I asked.

"As long as it doesn't cost him anything, or he doesn't get caught. I've heard neighbors claim that he doesn't milk a cow for two days before he takes her to the sales barn. That's so she'll look bagged full, like a heavy milker. I'm glad there aren't many like him."

"Me, too," I laughed, remembering how fragile he looked. "He seems so frail."

"Not Sol. He's tough and works hard. His shoes come off in early May and are forgotten until nearly October. Saves leather. I've seen him shovel graves barefooted. That takes special feet."

"Why is it that the poorest looking people seem to have the most money?" I said.

"You can count on it in this county," Elsie agreed, sliding into her coat.

On the back porch my visitor scrawled "Solomon Zimmerman" with a hesitant hand. He tore the check slowly from its binding. From previous encounters I doubted if our transaction was finished. He arose and shot a brown spurt into the flower bed at the edge of the porch.

"There now. Everything paid?" He unbuttoned a gray shirt cuff, grimy as a coal miner's. Pushing coat and shirt sleeve up a pipe-thin arm, he exposed loose wrinkled flesh. "See, no more rash," he gloated.

"That was more than eight years ago," I exclaimed, exasperated.

Sol knew this subject was an embarrassing episode in my career. We continued our game as I listened to my husband dish out stew and call the older children to supper.

Sol enjoyed reminding me of a wrong diagnosis during my first year of practice. Lizzie had visited my office complaining of nervousness and insomnia. We blamed her problems on a recent trip to Indiana by train. She and Sol rode coach, eating home-packed sandwiches and sleeping in their seats. They had moved among family and church friends for two weeks, with little time for rest.

Lizzie also showed me a scabby rash during her visit. She denied mosquitoes on their farm. I blamed it on her disturbed nerves.

At her next visit everything was improved but the rash, which seemed heavier than before. I dispensed a different ointment.

"Look at me now," she boasted several weeks later, raising heavy black skirts where the rash had been densest on her plump thighs. She removed her black bonnet so I could examine her neck at the edge of a white net cap. "See, no rash."

"The ointment worked," I said, pleased with the therapy.

"No, it wasn't the schmear. Sol had to go see old Doc Mentzer about some boils we couldn't cure with poultices. He had a rash, too. Doc said his rash looked like bites, and we should hunt around for bugs. When we lifted our mattress, bedbugs ran everywhere. They had a big nest under there. Guess we got them on the train."

"What did you do?" I asked, chagrined.

"Why, we had to move out of the house for several days. Henry's family lived in the barn, and we went to our son Harvey's while we hired a fumigator."

I considered the subject old and forgotten. "Have you and Lizzie taken any train rides lately?"

"No, not again," Sol laughed, putting away his checkbook and glasses. "I can't afford them. Only doctors can take vacations."

"Good-bye Sol," I called as he ambled off the porch and scuffed through fall leaves under the pear tree.

Sol untied his horse at the hitching rail in the backyard. He clucked at his bay and drove up the street. "See ya again, Kaiser."

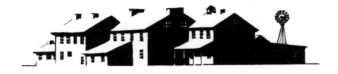

15.
Rain

"When the days get longer, the streams get stronger," a patient told me one fall when wells were dry. Springs had diminished to a trickle or stopped flowing, and many farmers hauled water to their stock, wandering the brown pastures.

The old lady was right. As the calendar passed December twenty-first and moved into winter, snows and rains became frequent. A northeaster could last a week, alternating between sheets of rain and a fine drizzle. At rare moments, the sun escaped the clouds long enough to prove it had not deserted earth forever.

Meadow dribbles became angry torrents covering roads and bridges with mud and debris. Most streams in eastern Lancaster County drained into the Conestoga creek, the Susquehanna river, and finally through barnyards, mired in ditches. I was scourged with ice and muck, and lashed with snow.

One early March storm, stream banks were full. I was

full too; full of dreary weather, tired of drying out wet children, of mud tracked through the house, and tired of the pile of dripping boots outside the door.

At bedtime I crawled under warm covers and listened to the rain beat the tin roof above our bedroom. Water slobbered over windows and gargled down the spouts. Wind scraped the old pear tree against the house and screeched skeleton branches across metal gutters. The weather stripping vibrated a chanting dirge.

Streams were still rising, and many roads would be impassable by morning. Three days of rain had washed the previous week's snow away to bare thawing ground. Weather forecasters saw no end of rain.

When Raymond Reiff called, it was not unexpected. I decided to wait at the Reiff home for Martha to deliver. Pulling on boots, raincoat, and plastic bandana, I set out for Shaum's Corner.

The windshield wipers beat at full speed. New Holland Pike was not flooded, but on Newport Road toward Brownstown, water lay in the low places and streams raced before my headlights like rivers. Overloaded culverts heaped weeds against fences and piled debris on the macadam. Bridges became dams and meadows lakes.

It was comforting to see taillights several blocks ahead. At Talmage I stopped at the edge of a swirling stream of unknown depth and several car-lengths' width, a meadow trickle gone wild. It would be miles farther to drive around by another route; probably no better, and possibly worse. The taillights ahead continued. I shifted into low gear, held a steady slow speed, and started across. Water came to the door, and the exhaust sputtered like a motorboat.

On the other side I tested the brakes. Nothing. I crawled

through Talmage and Brownstown to Shaum's Corner, pumping the brakes until they began to hold, then pulled to one side and finally stopped at the highway to Lancaster.

A large branch of the Conestoga creek lay ahead. I crossed the concrete bridge onto a side road. It ran several hundred feet along the stream before leaving the flood plain and higher ground. The creek had spilled over its banks but was still a foot below the roadway.

On the Reiff lane, snow tires pulled the car through submerged mire, axle deep. I rode the tracks, turning the wheel in the direction the car was skidding.

Martha and Raymond's kitchen was warm and comfortable. I was glad that this Mennonite family had a telephone in their house so I would not have to run out through the rain to the car if I had any messages.

Raymond, in faded jeans and brown plaid flannel shirt, sat in a recliner with ankle-high work shoes propped on the footrest. Martha, wrapped in a blue terry cloth bathrobe and crocheted footwarmers, paced the flowered linoleum several hours while we talked about coming spring work, how high the streams had risen in past years, how high they might be tomorrow.

We spoke softly so we would not wake the sleeping family upstairs or the cribbed toddler, pushed from the bedroom into the parlor for the night.

Martha's labor was progressing well, and she showed signs of impending delivery when my husband telephoned. Sol Beiler, 25 miles away, had called asking me to come to Mount Eden. His wife was in labor. He thought it wise if I came soon because of the weather.

It was impossible to leave Martha now. I asked Pete to call Sol back at his pay phone and say that I would come as soon as possible. Naomi should relax until I could get to the Beiler home.

Martha was in her final stage of delivery when a second call came. Sol asked me to hurry. I promised arrival at Beilers in an hour. Even in the rain I should be able to manage. I crossed my fingers.

A few minutes later Martha's new son lay bundled at her side. Hurriedly, I gave postpartum instructions, left the cleanup work to Raymond, and ran out the walk. The storm seemed to be in remission.

I turned the key in the ignition. The starter whirred furiously. The engine was dead. I pumped the accelerator. Tried again. The deep stream at Talmage, I thought. Expert at changing tires, I knew nothing about drying a soggy engine. The Reiffs drove a horse. It was between midnight and dawn.

On the third try the reluctant engine started, gasped, died, started again. The car sputtered forward, not all cylinders working. I reasoned that the motor would heat up and dry out if it ran long enough.

The car hesitated several times down the mucky lane, threatening to die. I moved in spasms to the hard road.

Driving downhill to the floodplain, I could see that the water had risen over the edge of the road. Sticks, floating brush, and several tin cans bumped along the macadam like chickens pecking corn at feeding time. In the headlight, a tree surged rapidly downstream. If the water rose another foot the road would be impassable, and owners of summer cottages along the banks would spend vacations shoveling mud from porches and interiors.

Halfway to the bridge the car sputtered and jerked to a stop. The creek roared along in the dark like a waterfall. I turned the key. Nothing. I twisted it again. The engine stammered and died. Another turn and it roared an off-beat. The car crawled across the bridge to Shaum's Corner, less than a mile from the Reiff home.

Near the corner, the car again became perverse and died. The old skating rink, now an empty apartment house, seemed to watch with a cold unsympathetic stare. Its rain-streaked crumbling plaster suited the mood of the desolate night as I tried to coax life into a wet engine. Finally, I jerked forward and onto the highway to Lancaster.

The well-traveled concrete ribbon passed through fields edged with houses and crossroad villages. On a rain-soaked night it was deserted. At Sandy Ridge I became hopeful. I had traveled about four miles, was on higher ground, and believed my troubles were over. Then the engine died again . . . permanently. With the last inertia, the station wagon drifted onto a lane. No amount of persuasion could spark another response from the drowned motor.

The gravel lane clung to the wheels and stopped them. Half on the highway, the station wagon was too heavy to push farther in the doughy lane. The silhouetted house beside the driveway was dark.

Headlights shone over the hill to the north. Running lights of a tractor-trailer rig came toward me, fast. "Good-bye, Ambassador wagon," I muttered and ran down the highway, wildly waving both arms.

The driver saw me as I jumped to the berm. With an explosion of air brakes, the bob-tailed tractor stopped several feet short of the protruding station wagon.

A round-bellied man in leather jacket and cap jumped to the road and walked toward me through the steady rain.

"Drowned out," he said, smiling.

My luck had changed. He laughed as I explained the urgency of babies and time and rain-washed roads. Putting a burly shoulder to the car, he pushed it into the driveway as if it were a toy express wagon.

"I'm on my way home to Lancaster," he said. "Just left my trailer of goods at a distribution center in Ephrata. Can I take ya into the city?"

"Great," I answered. Someone at the hospital in Lancaster could probably lend me a car to finish the trip.

Dripping water from coat and scarf, loose hair hanging in strings around my face, I set a note on the dashboard of the crippled station wagon for the owners of the borrowed lane, picked up my bag, and clambered into the high cab beside the good Samaritan. He was busy devouring a large chocolate bar.

"Don't worry about your muddy boots. Can't keep nothin' clean or dry this weather," he said, smiling. His coarse round face, framed by kinky red hair, shoved his greasy cap to a rakish angle. A bushy beard of the same color trapped rain drops and reflected light from the dash like a lit Christmas tree.

Apparently glad for company on a wet night, he chatted as if hungry for a listener. Between bites of his candy bar he chain-smoked until the air was a blue haze. I became sleepy in the warm dry cab.

Truck drivers had a reputation for friendliness, for helping the helpless along highways. But another fear began to gnaw into my newfound comfort. The unfamiliar truck, riding the night with a stranger . . . I refused his chocolate and set my black bag between us.

At the same time I was infinitely grateful to my rescuer. I wrote his Lancaster address on a prescription pad and resolved to send him a gift of appreciation, should life ever dry out and return to normal.

By the time we reached Lancaster, the ride and my stubby friend had become a pleasure. Rain and fresh air hit me like a slap on the face as I descended the cab at Cottage and East Orange streets. "Thank you, thank you," I repeated profusely.

Using my key, I entered the hospital through the doctor's entrance and went to a telephone in the lounge to call the night intern. No transportation there. His wife had driven him to work, and the doctor on call had no car. At intern quarters Bayer James was the only car owner, but no one was joyful about night calls.

I was desperate and knew Bayer well. He had often assisted at my delivery table and had visited my home and office. I did not doubt his willingness to go with me. It was his car I doubted. I could not drive the temperamental critter myself.

Bayer had a love affair with a revitalized Model A Ford. He kept its gray body waxed to a high shine and drove it everywhere. They seemed a good team: trim, jaunty, carefree, and not caring if they got to a place or not. Could I depend upon this matched pair?

Tonight there was no choice. How could I take a taxi to Mount Eden? How could I afford a taxi if one would consent to drive me? What took Bayer so long to come to the phone?

"Yes, I'll come. I'll take you," his sleepy voice finally answered.

Time no longer counted. The promised hour was long past. All I could hope was that Naomi would be slower than she predicted and would remain undelivered.

My driver gloated. His Model A was in demand when my car had expired. He expounded affectionately upon the advantages of owning a vintage model.

Bayer's loose rumpled raincoat fit the occasion. He jammed an Irish tweed hat on his head. "Just the thing to shed rain," he laughed. From an inner pocket he pulled a scarred Briar and filled the cup with the sweet odor of pipe tobacco.

We bounced through the downpour to a rhythm only Model A Fords can produce. I clutched my bag while peering through the fogged windshield to give directions and watch for water on the roads. A handful of gauze pads, wiped across the windshield, reduced the mist. Sometimes I could have run as fast as we drove.

"I've never seen a home birth. What are they like?" Bayer asked, leaning forward and scowling to see through the rain.

"Oh, I just pull on a pair of rubber gloves and catch the baby," I said with a glib shrug. "This is number 12 for Naomi. Let's hope we make it in time to catch this one."

"Sorry, this car won't go any faster."

"Hope everything is okay. I don't remember Naomi's name on this month's delivery list, but I don't keep them all in my head."

East of Strasburg we climbed out of the valley to higher ground, and travel became easier. Near Mount Eden we parked between the Beiler's house and barn. Dim light cast pale shafts into the night from around the edges of window shades in a corner room. No one met us at the back door. By my waning flashlight we floundered up the broken concrete walk and into a cavernous kitchen, barely lit by a small kerosene lamp on a long table.

"Where are you?" I called.

"Better get in here," Sol answered from a distant room.

We ran through the kitchen, down a hall to streaks of light beneath a door.

"What kept you?" Naomi looked at us between knees flexed above the mattress.

"You're late. See what we have." Sol nodded proudly toward a pile of moving blankets beside Naomi. In a calloused hand, he held two limp umbilical cords tied with grocery store string.

Stunned, I stared at the swarthy gray-bearded Amishman standing beside his wife. "Don't pull on them," I said, feeling a desperate need to say something important.

"Twin girls. Both bottom-end first," Sol boasted. "Both cried right away. Both fine and almost a month early. Good thing I watched you deliver a few others. You sure missed this time." Stocking-footed, he stepped back on the linoleum to allow me to deliver the placenta.

The word "breech" always filled me with apprehension. Sol had just delivered two.

"I'll have to get you to deliver all my upside-downers," I teased as the placenta slid into a wash basin.

Sol slipped boots over his work-a-day broadfalls and went into the drizzle to bury the placenta in the manure pile at the barn.

I gave Naomi a clean dry bed and dressed the babies. Bayer examined them before we put them to breast.

"Not bad for a 42-year-old," Naomi chuckled. "Never thought I'd ever have twins. Won't the other children be surprised!"

Bayer drove me home to New Holland. We staggered across country, wiping the windshield and circumventing engorged streams. He still had not seen a home delivery, but I knew everyone at the hospital would hear about this night. They would hear the merits of owning an old car.

I never sent a bill for my trip to Mount Eden, nor was I paid. "We'll chalk that night up to experience," I told Sol.

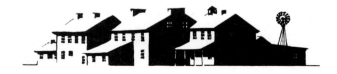

16.
On a Mattress

"**B**ut what shall I do? Where can I go?" Marjorie Riley cried. Tears filled her big blue eyes and rolled over round cheeks onto the beaded peasant blouse. "What do I do now?" She patted the head of a frightened toddler hanging firmly to her gingham skirt.

The child, on seeing her mother cry, turned down the corners of a trembling mouth and wailed. She was dressed like Marjorie in blouse and long skirt. Grimy sandaled feet hopped about on her mother's sandals.

"I'm sorry," I said, handing her a tissue from a box perched on a pile of medical journals beside my desk. "Millersville is too far out of my usual territory."

Marjorie wiped her eyes and the baby's pug nose. "Emma Fisher, where we buy sweet corn, said that you deliver women at home even if they aren't Amish. She said you would help us. Michael works after college and weekends at a gas station. We'll pay you." Tears ran over the freckles that bridged her nose and winged toward ears hidden by hair yellow as spring honey. She pulled fussing Peggy onto her lap.

"No," I said gently but firmly. "It would be bad enough to drive 25 miles, but going through Lancaster City makes it impossible. It isn't fair to my closer patients who might need me. I could care for you if you came halfway to the hospital."

"Please come to Millersville. We want our baby at home. Please," she begged, dabbing her eyes with the soggy tissue. She began to cry again. "We'll even pay you extra. There isn't any doctor in Millersville who delivers babies at home."

I slowly shook my head. "No." Could she sense me softening? If she had only pleaded her case over the telephone where I could not see her distress. Marjorie was the age of my older daughter. I would want someone to help her if she needed it. Several times I had traveled 25 miles or even farther.

"Michael and I want to be together for the whole labor and delivery. No crowd of doctors and nurses running around everywhere; no pills or shots." She ran slender fingers through waistlength tresses. She dropped her eyes like a whipped puppy.

"Well, all right," I agreed with a sigh, reaching for a blank patient record. "If I agree to come to your home it will be a gamble." Could I believe my own words? "If a patient closer to New Holland should need me, you must go to the hospital."

Marjorie became sunshine. She sniffed, mopped her eyes, gleamed the innocent child-smile that had won me. "Thank you. Thank you. We'll take that chance." She comforted sniffling Peggy. "We're happy now. Everything will be okay."

As I picked up a pen to begin the history and physical, I wondered if I would regret my decision. I pondered how a general might feel after losing a battle. I had given battle and allowed myself to be defeated by a girl armed with tears and sincerity.

All summer I saw Marjorie and Peggy regularly. If not pumping gas, Michael came with them. His lean, six-foot body moved quickly as he dived to snatch Peggy from mischief or balanced her wiggling body on an arm. A stack of untamable red hair topped his ruddy thin face. His rusty beard made him appear 10 years older than his exuberant wife. At times we became knotted in his breathless nonstop strings of questions. He read everything he could find about childbirth and quizzed me in detail. If I could not get to their home when needed, I knew by mutual understanding that he intended to deliver his bulging spouse himself.

Marjorie took pregnancy seriously. She attributed her healthful glow to exercise, tofu, and a vegetarian diet. Anxiously, she awaited the birth, wanting perfection. I, too, was caught up in her zest for life: her own, the baby she carried, and everyone around her. By the time she reached term our family was known to her by name, habits, and interests.

On a Saturday in late September, smelling of fall and dank from Friday night's frost, Marjorie called me to Millersville. Sumac and gum trees soared red along country roadbanks. The topmost maple branches were capped with new gold.

Lancaster City was busy with weekend traffic, and I hoped my patient had allowed enough time for me to reach her. Millersville Pike was not much better, but George Street was quiet as I passed the old college, once Millersville Normal School. I turned onto a side street and parked behind a semi-detached brick house stained dark by time.

An uneven concrete walk divided the backyard into two vegetable gardens. I walked past frost-brown tomato plants sagged with green nubbins clinging stubbornly to gaunt stalks. Rows of intermittent cabbages hugged the earth like teeth in a Halloween pumpkin. Fern-topped carrots and burnished beet leaves marked the year's last harvests.

In the small kitchen, my patient worked before scarred wooden cupboards and a knicked porcelain sink. A stringy width of flowered muslin barely concealed a box of pots and pans under the sink. Along one wall a freezer hummed an incessant monotone.

Marjorie was setting a batch of yogurt to culture in the oven of a rusted chipped gas stove. Peggy hung on her skirts or scampered barefoot between kitchen and living rom.

"Come in. Glad to see you," Marjorie said. She had gambled and won. Triumph shone in her wide smile. I compared her even white teeth to our daughter's and wondered if Marjorie's parents had paid more or less orthodontist fees than we had. They had gotten their money's worth I thought. She smiled at everything all the time. Nothing seemed to worry Marjorie. I remembered our first meeting. Had those tears been honest ones?

It seemed many years since my college days. The mother's attic/grandma's cellar decor of school-life apartments seemed lost in cobwebbed memories until I followed Marjorie's bare feet through the sparsely furnished living room into the bedroom.

Michael sat at a desk surrounded by papers and books, rumpling his kinky hair with thick fingers as he wrote homework. He stopped only to turn a page or scratch an ear while he concentrated.

"Hello, see you made it," Michael said. Removing a pencil from his mouth, he leaned back and watched me search the room.

"Oh! Uh—I forgot to tell you," Marjorie sputtered with a guilty grin. She, too, watched me. Was she afraid I surely would not have come if I had known what I now saw?

Surprises were not new, but this! "We don't have a regular bed," she laughed.

There was no bed in the frugal room. Beyond Peggy's rickety crib, a mattress lay in a corner on the bare floor. It was sheeted, properly covered, and prepared according to instructions.

On a scarred mahogany bureau, baby garments, a basin, baby scales, and clean cloths were laid out in neat piles. I had not specified any particular kind of bed. Must a bed be off the floor, I asked myself.

Michael slid down into his chair, smiled, and watched me examine his wife when she nimbly laid on the mattress.

I wiggled a glove onto a hand and bent from the waist to examine Marjorie. Possible, but awkward. An unprofessional stance at best. I squatted on my haunches beside her. Ungraceful, as well as unstable and uncomfortable. Next, I knelt on my knees. Decidedly the most workable choice.

"Your baby is coming down nicely," I told them. "However, it faces up toward Marjorie's abdomen instead of looking toward her back. Usually not serious. Perhaps a longer labor."

"Don't interfere! No shots!" Michael shouted. He sat upright, folded his arms across his chest and pulled nervously at his beard.

"What can I do to help?" Marjorie asked, rising to sit cross-legged on the mattress. She was without a smile.

"Knee-chest position helps sometimes," I answered, glad to resume an upright position. "Usually they rotate without help. Babies can deliver face up."

Michael seemed satisfied that no dangerous or heroic maneuver was about to occur. He returned to his studies until time to join his wife on the mattress.

Marjorie entertained Peggy until her labor became stronger. She rose from the floor with ease and changed into one of Michael's shirts, wearing it backward, unbuttoned. She began Lamaze breathing.

After arranging my obstetrical equipment and explaining each item, I took a copy of *Good Housekeeping* from my bag. It was luxury reading, for medical journals piled higher and higher beside my desk. Guilt and dwindling space pushed me to them when I had free time at home. In the middle of the room I found a comfortable chair beside an old oak table.

Before uncurtained windows, Peggy climbed a frayed plush sofa or slid down a worn upholstered armchair. She collided several times with a floor lamp, sending its heat-stained shade across the room. Tired of that game, she went to a Maltese cat asleep on the braided rug. Baby-jabber brought no response but a thrust of toes to its stomach sent tabby to higher ground atop a stereo.

My senses were divided between an exotic garden salad and the wonders of flower art when Marjorie called me to check her. I knelt, examined, arose, and returned to the chair many times, ignoring my snapping joints which I imagined could be heard on the front street. My hips and legs began to tire.

"Soon?" Marjorie asked between pants. She smiled.

"Very soon now," I answered. "The baby has rotated just fine." It would not be too soon for me.

Michael sat cross-legged on the mattress with his back against the wall. He cradled Marjorie's head and shoulders on his knees as he coached her labor.

"Remember how to breathe. Push. Breathe. Relax. It's soon here," Michael said.

I lost count of ups and downs; they became more frequent and lasted longer. This was a mattress party.

Michael's muscular arms supported Marjorie as she worked. He held his breath when she did, tensed and pushed with her. His calloused, grease-stained hands wrung out wet washcloths to cool her neck and face. Between contractions they laughed about the good times they would have with their new son.

I shifted weight frequently, winced as a mattress button pressed into a knee. Michael seemed amused and laughed that I should be uncomfortable on the floor mattress.

"Our baby's nearly here!" Marjorie called to Peggy who danced and jumped in her crib above our heads.

Peggy's strawberry curls bounced as she rattled the crib sides and fired toys onto the floor. "Baby. Baby," she shouted.

"Come on Margie. Push hard." Michael's face contorted with effort.

Wet hair on the baby's scalp began to show on the perineum. At each contraction more black appeared until the head was born. I aspirated mucus from the nose, awaited Marjorie's next contraction, and a fat baby lay on the mattress.

"Another girl," Michael shouted. "Suits me."

"Let me see her. Let me have my baby." Marjorie was laughing, hyper, excited. She raised her arms to her new daughter.

The baby whimpered and grunted as I laid her on Marjorie's chest. The newborn brushed the breast several times, rooted, then began to nurse as if suckling were her reason for birth.

While the baby warmed under blankets from a hot radiator, the cord stopped pulsing. I cut it and delivered the placenta. There were no injections, no sutures, little cleaning up.

Ahhh. It was time to rise from the mattress for the last time. I stood up slowly, testing each muscle.

If one afternoon on a mattress made me stiff and sore, I pondered how I would manage old age.

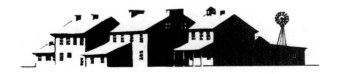

17.
Barn of Money

If it had not been for Ezra Miller's new cow, I doubt if I would have raised my obstetrical fee that year.

Charges were a touchy part of medical practice. Even if I had donated my services, a few patients would have dickered about costs. The ragged farmer who owned three farms grumbled the most.

Older patients boasted of babies costing only 10 or 15 dollars during the Great Depression. When I began practice in 1951, 75 dollars was a reasonable birthing fee, and three dollars covered an office visit. Charges increased with time and the rising economy.

Money was not on my mind the Saturday in January I made a house call at Ezra Miller's farm. Winter was granting a welcome recess from cold and storms. The warmth of the sun on bare cheeks gave a sure promise of spring, but a lingering chill kept outdoorsmen buttoned in their coats.

Ezra's wife Feeny, Pennsylvania Dutch nickname for Lavina, had been confined to bed several weeks, threatening to miscarry an early pregnancy. This was not new to Feeny, who had several miscarriages before she had learned that bed rest was justified. Healthy full-term babies, delivered in the bed that now imprisoned her, made weeks of inactivity worthwhile.

Feeny had expected me on Friday, but the call was not urgent, and there had been no other visits in the area. Besides, I expected my brother and his wife Virginia for the weekend. Recently retired from the Navy, John was now engaged in planting an orchard and truck farming.

A drive through the farm country would be an ideal way to entertain my guests. We had been reared on a small Pennsylvania farm similar to the Lancaster County ones with their massive bank barns and imposing two-story farmhouses.

Virginia, a tall woman with dignity and charm, slid in beside me in the station wagon. John folded himself in beside her and stuffed his legs under the dashboard.

We drove eastward through New Holland and descended into the crossroad town of Blue Ball and past its historic hotel with a blue ball dangling above its door.

Ascending the next ridge we traveled the shoestring towns of Goodville and then Churchtown, named for its many houses of worship in Colonial days.

The country was patched with small farms falling away from the highway ridge on both sides. It gave us a clear view into valleys of fallow acres, fields of corn shocks, and green splotches of winter wheat.

This part of the county, once deeded to Welsh settlers under a William Penn land grant, had many years ago been divided and subdivided into small farms now owned by Amish and Mennonites.

On a bright afternoon there was activity in the fields. Brawny work horses hauled manure spreaders over the frozen ground or pulled wagon loads of fodder, shocked after last fall's cornhusking, into barns.

Housewives, dressed in coats, galoshes, and bonnets, planted hotbeds for early lettuce and garden seedlings. We saw jacketed girls raking leaves from under yard bushes, their heads covered with colorful bandanas.

Near Morgantown the tall smokestacks of Bethlehem Steel jutted like a monument above the deep mines. It contrasted the squat farmhouse chimneys in the Conestoga Valley.

We stopped twice at mailboxes along our route to deliver medications. I performed this service often when on calls. Elva Zeiset had mailed a note, written on the back of December's calendar page, asking me to "drop off" the prenatal vitamins she forgot at her last office visit. Harvey Zimmerman, usually absent-minded, had telephoned to renew his supply of digitalis.

"How will they know you've been here?" Virginia asked. "Don't your packages get mixed up with the mail?"

"I thought it is illegal to use the mailboxes," John said.

"Hold your ears and watch," I said, blasting the horn several times.

Elva, at the other end of the long lane, ran into the yard and waved her apron vigorously. I beeped and waved back.

Harvey opened his front door and bellowed, "Okay," between cupped hands.

"I couldn't possibly deliver these packages to the doors. I'd be invited into each house for long conversations or detailed free consultations. No day would be long enough."

"Medical practice is sure different in the country," John laughed, shaking his head.

"Local drugstores renew prescriptions by mail or phone for horse-and-buggy people. Sometimes the pharmacist sets the package on the bus. The recipient meets the bus to pick up his medication and mails a check to the pharmacy," I explained to my amazed guests.

We passed the stone quarry on Maxwell's Hill and turned onto the Miller lane, flanked on each side by a deep ditch, a whitewashed board fence, and a row of knobby maples.

"Watch it!" Virginia cried. "We'll hit the barn."

I made a quick right turn on the lane or we would have driven up the barn bridge, through the wide sliding doors, and onto the barn floor above the stables.

Virginia and John inspected the gray canvas Amish market wagon in the driveway while I went to the house.

"Who's with you?" Ezra asked, putting down the morning paper. He rose from the rolling desk chair at his end of the kitchen table and nudged several children from the windows.

"My brother and his wife. They like farms." I hoped he would invite them into the house and felt certain he would.

"Bring them in. Where do they live?" Ezra went to the door and waved my guests through the washhouse into the kitchen.

The Amish are well aware of outsiders' interest in their homes and culture. Some kitchens are modern and convenient. The Millers' was old-fashioned. I had forewarned my companions to observe this Amish kitchen with its many decorative calendars of various months and years, the old stove, but mostly the hospitality of the people.

"You don't have a cookstove like this one," Ezra said, pointing to the black Majestic.

"No, but I like your beautiful woodwork," Virginia said, looking at the cupboards and running a hand over the dark-stained wainscoting. It covered the walls from chair rail to floor.

"Hand-combed," Ezra explained. "Been here for years. Combed graining like that used to be a specialty. None of our people do it anymore. We expect to remodel soon."

"What a pity," Virginia said.

"Makes the kitchen too dark. We'll tear out that old boarded up fireplace in the corner, too. Give us more room. Sell the cookstove with its ashes and dust."

"What will you cook on?" John asked.

"The gas stove. We use it only in summer now. The space heaters will keep us warm enough."

"Do I hear water dripping?" Virginia asked.

"Yes. We'll get rid of this, too," Ezra said, opening a wide cupboard door in the wall between the kitchen and washhouse. "Not many of these left. We've had a gas refrigerator for years; just keep extras in this trough. A door on the other side opens into the kettlehouse, the washhouse."

In the space between the walls, water ran in spasms into a zinc-lined trough. An overflow pipe carried water to the barn. A crock of milk, a quart of pickles, and a jar of applesauce sat in the flowing water. Above them on shelves sat dishes of butter and jelly and a bowl of chocolate pudding.

"The waterwheel down at the creek pumps water from the well beside the house into this trough," Ezra said, offering a drink of the water from an enamel cup hanging on a nail in the compartment.

"We'll wait until next winter to tear everything up," Ezra smiled shyly. "It makes too much fuss with Feeny in bed. Anyway, it's soon time for spring plowing."

"Have a cookie?" Ezra's oldest daughter, age 15, asked. She removed a hot tray from the range oven and put a new batch to bake.

The big kitchen was filled with the aroma of chocolate chip cookies stacked on the table. When we each accepted one, it seemed a signal for the five children shadowing our movements to taste also. Big sister smiled benevolently.

"Save some for Mam," she said, laughing.

Feeny waited for me in the bedroom off the kitchen. "How much longer in this bed?" she asked hopefully. "My elbows are sore from rubbing the sheets."

She looked frail and thin lying under a blue dahlia quilt. Her small face against the white bolster seemed pale from the weeks of confinement. Wisps of sandy hair escaped her muslin nightcap and long braids.

"We'll see," I said opening my bag. I trickled a dab of conductive jelly on her belly and moved the doppler above her pubis. Gurgling and rumbling sounds came through the microphone. Then a fair "tic, a-tic, a-tic, a-tic" in regular rhythm.

"The baby's heartbeat. I'm so glad." Feeny's face brightened. "I want to meet your sister-in-law, but not your brother. Don't want any strange men seeing me in bed."

"Hearing the heartbeat sure cheered you up."

"Yup. Makes staying in bed easier. It's time for another baby around here. Amanda's past two." Feeny smiled, showing small white teeth.

I nodded. Children are not only loved and wanted but necessary on a farm. They are its strength, life, and perpetuity.

Feeny quizzed Virginia about her children, Connecticut life, whether her parents were living, their ages, the price of her paisley print dress.

Virginia's eyes wandered over the high sleigh-backed bed, the oak chest of drawers, nails hung with clothing along one wall, windowsills of geraniums and coleus, brightly colored needlepoint cushions on the rocking chairs.

"We're going to the barn. Want to go along?" John called.

Eager to see as much of the farm as possible, Virginia joined the expedition.

I finished my visit with Feeny and went to find the tour. Under the barn forebay, I passed the concrete watering trough. Last summer goldfish had threaded through its mossy depths. They had fed on grain washed from the horses' mouths. Today thick ice clouded the winter trough.

The four children, three adults, and two mongrel sheep dogs were not in the cow stable. Barns produced nostalgic memories for me of my childhood spent on a small Bucks County farm. I remembered the half dozen Jersey, Guernsey, and Holstein cows in Father's meager stable. We hand-milked them twice a day, carried the foaming buckets to a small milkhouse and strained the milk into cans, cooling in a cement water trough.

"Hello," I called walking past the cows. The scent of sweet hay, the crisp yellow straw, the quiet breathing seemed comfortable and cozy.

"These are my four mules," Ezra explained when I found the entourage at the far side of the barn. "I also keep two field horses and a driving horse for the carriage."

"And a pony," my brother said, pointing a scrawny finger toward the trim little animal in a corner stall.

"That's for the kids. Mom drives it with the cart sometimes."d

"Look here," Samuel, a boy about 10, said. He walked to a pile of hay. "These kittens are only three weeks old."

Each mewing baby was passed around until all six were admired. The tabby seemed happy when her family of spots, stripes, and calico was returned to the nest. Cats are an important part of barn life, keeping the rat and mice population under control. I do not remember ever seeing a cat as an Amish house pet.

We stopped at the calf pen a moment to pet the black and whites. They nuzzled our fingers or jumped from our reach. Ten future milkers shared a large pen.

Ezra and John talked nonstop.

"How old are you?" Ezra asked.

"Thirty-nine. And you?"

"The same."

There the similarity ended. Ezra, short and stumpy, appeared nearly neckless under his beard and dusty black broadbrim. His home-sewn black jacket, relegated for farm work, was tattered, and the broadfall pants were neatly patched and repatched. A brown bristly beard covered half a dark face. The chest-length whiskers moved in snappy vibrations as he emphasized sentences.

The farmer's nose was a round blob set between rounder cheeks. His rotund figure did not prevent him from jumping around the stable as if the floor were charged with electricity.

John, six foot three, had to bend over in order to speak with Ezra who barely came to his shoulder. My brother was cleanshaven with a long face, emphasizing his long neck and lean body. He listened quietly to Ezra, resting one cheek in the palm of his hand.

"Is that a fact?" John drawled several times, furrowing his high forehead as Ezra piped the facts of farming. It was all he found time to say.

They did share a violent gesturing with their hands. John flailed Ichabod arms and aimed bony fingers. Ezra waved short arms and pointed stubby digits at imaginary objects.

The Miller children watched, mute for a long time, not understanding the conversation. Finally, little girls of two and four tore their wool scarves from pigtailed heads, threw black jackets on a straw pile, and raced tricycles around the cemented cow stable.

Samuel climbed up the silo to throw down ensilage (fermented chopped corn) for the cows' supper.

"I'm eight," Salome told Virgina. The child lingered to talk about her one-room school and how she washed dishes and helped in the house and around the barn.

My sister-in-law was entranced by the little girl with pigtails wrapped around her head and dressed in Amish clothing. Salome was equally captivated by the importance of her conversation with a woman from the world outside her plain community.

"See that plastic pipe," Ezra said. Hopping onto a straw bale, he pointed to a white line running the length of the stable along the ʳ ʲugh-timbered ceiling. "That tube takes milk from the cows to the bulk cooler in the milkhouse."

Ezra jumped the ditch behind a big white cow. "Milk never touches my hands." He gave the cow an affectionate smack on the rump and leaped across the gutter where we stood between two rows of swinging tails.

We admired the 32 head of milk producers stanchioned between a drainage ditch and the concrete feed trough under their noses.

"How can you use milkers?" John asked. "I don't see any electricity."

"Milking and cooling are done by a diesel engine."

"You don't say," John pointed to an arc of wire suspended above the rump of each cow. "What are they?"

"Oh, that," Ezra laughed. "They keep the cow from humping so all the manure lands in the ditch. It gives a small shock if she touches it. Not many farmers have them. Storage batteries give the charge, like the pasture fence."

"Is it that you don't use electricity from the lines along the road?" Virginia asked.

Ezra gave a quick nod and went on to explain how the cows draw water into iron bowls beside them by pushing their noses against a lever.

"This fine herd must represent a lot of money," Virginia said, scanning the rows of cows.

"A cow costs plenty." The farmer eyed his Holsteins with pride. "Daisy over there cost 600 dollars, Blacky here was 700 three years ago, Maggie 500."

"Is that a fact?" John said.

"They're all good stock. I keep production records on each one. A few men still keep bulls, but most have gone to artificial insemination. Feeny keeps track of those things in her diary, along with planting and other dates."

John wrinkled his brows, mentally calculating the financial investment in the stable.

"Oh yes," Ezra continued, "vets aren't any cheaper than doctors." He laughed at me with eyes twinkling.

I ignored his bait and pretended to hear none of the conversation or the gibe.

"Now that big cow over there," Ezra motioned toward a large cow with scattered black patches across her rump. She chewed her cud in a corner stall. Late afternoon sunshine, reflecting off the whitewashed stone walls of the barn through a tier of high windows, gave her coat a sheen nearly iridescent. Her stance was noble and erect. "That's a new milker. Paid 900 for her. I expect good milk production and fine calves. She's fresh. Some men pay 1,200 for a top cow."

The talk during the remainder of the tour scarcely registered with me. I had heard many times that farm profits lay in growing as much feed grain as possible, that feed was too high. Dairy company inspectors were strict and finicky, demanding. Low milk prices were not new either, but the cost of cows . . .

My fee for a baby birthing would not cast a shadow on the expense of buying a cow. Wrapped in thoughts of expenditures, profits, and benefits, I followed the group as we left the warmth of the stable to inspect the bulk milk tank, a stainless steel monster with stirring paddle and gauges. A row of milkers hung like four-legged spiders from a rack. The milkhouse was acrid with disinfectant.

"We heat our water with propane gas. See that big tank beside the barn? It supplies the stove and refrigerator in the house, too." Ezra pulled a leather thong from a pants pocket and looked at his pocket watch. "Time to get started with the evening work."

Our expedition was finished. Ezra, the three girls, and two woolly dogs walked to the car with us. The men still discussed farming.

I had made a decision. The present maternity fee seemed too little in light of the economy around me. Monday morning I hung a new notice in my waiting room.

AS OF FEB. 1st, 1974
ALL NEW OBSTETRICAL CASES
$175.00

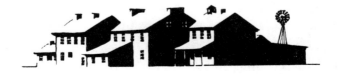

18.
Blizzard

Everyone watched for the first flakes.

The storm, conceived in the Gulf of Mexico, labored northeast as a blizzard. It bore across Georgia, the Carolinas, and into Virginia.

The South lay swathed in snow. Highways closed, isolating entire towns as violence pushed up the coast. By noon it had arrived in Wilmington, an hour's drive south of Lancaster.

Since the day before, a dense cloud cover, gray as an oyster shell, drifted across January skies in fitful streaks. Moisture-laden air hovered below freezing. It penetrated the heaviest clothing with chilling discomfort.

After lunch I delivered a pre-storm baby, glad for one less birth to worry about during a blizzard. I hurried through the countryside finishing rounds to patients who might be isolated for several days.

Along the roads, people scurried to prepare for the storm. Farmers hauled extra fodder from fields into barns.

They spread manure on fields and carried ensilage from outdoor trenches to cattle. Housewives made hurried trips to grocery stores. Trucks, cars, and buggies, rushing on last minute errands, congested the highways.

Driving home through Hatville, I saw the first snow, a fine dust like baby powder. I remembered Grandfather and his recollections of the '88 blizzard. He said the sure sign of a big storm was one which began with small flakes.

Within minutes, the snow fell in a frenzy covering everything. It changed fence posts and bushes into smeared shadows. Clouds closed in, shrinking visibility to a few yards. Travel was slow and tedious on slippery roads.

When I finally arrived home, Gertrude Glick, our eight-to-four housekeeper had a foot in one galosh and stomped the second shoe into the other. Her black coat lay over a chair.

"Looks like the real thing out there," Gertie said, without her usual smile. "I better go buy bread and milk if there's any left." She pulled a black bonnet over her net cap, wrapped a muffler around her neck, and kissed the children. "See you when I can get here again."

The supper odor of liver and onions still hung in the air, mingling with puffs of smoke from the fireplace when the telephone rang.

"This is Martin Weaver. Guess you better come out. We think Martha's in labor."

"How are your roads?"

"Ours is drifted shut, but Shirk Road is still open. I'll meet you at the corner in half an hour with the carriage and drive ya in."

"Okay, I'll start now." I could not hide my lack of enthusiasm.

"Too bad I have to baby-sit," Pete said. His grin meant "Glad it's not me."

"Lucky you," I grumbled, regretting the day I chose to become a doctor.

I telephoned Anna. During her years in the office, she went on home births with me. It was often helpful to have an extra pair of hands.

The wind whistled around our old farmhouse. Gusts blew smoke down the chimney, giving the house a woodsy fragrance. I envied my husband reading before the burning logs.

No choice. Pulling on long underwear, I comforted myself with the thought that this call could have been a 13-mile trip instead of three.

"Keep the bed warm." I wrinkled my nose at Pete, pulled a hood over the wool hat and slammed the door, hoping the cold draft would penetrate his conscience.

The thermometer read 15 degrees. I threw a shovel into the station wagon. Any thoughts of an easy trip whirled away with the white powder which blew in clouds across the road and dimmed the street lights.

Down the block I pulled curbside, blew the horn, and waited for Anna. An icy blast rushed her along the sidewalk. Swathed in a knobby red coat, fur hat, and green plaid muffler, she tumbled onto the front seat.

"What a night. Think we'll have to walk?" she asked through mist that fogged her glasses. She stamped her boots, knocking snow into the car.

"No walking tonight. We get a carriage ride," I said, shifting gears and peering through the storm.

The laboring storm hit us full impact at the borough line where the last street light guarded New Holland.

Unprotected by houses, giant drifts usually piled up and isolated those on the inside from the rest of the world.

We made our escape through deepening mounds until we reached Shirk Road. Snow eddies attacked from every side. Writhing gusts shook the station wagon. In places the road was bare; in others I gunned the engine and we flew through downy tunnels.

I recalled these same roadbanks last spring, overgrown with violets, wild mustard, and dandelion, the air perfumed with honeysuckle.

"The side roads will soon be drifted shut," Anna said.

'This one is shut now." I stopped on the crest of a hill.

Our headlights shone across a valley of shifting snow. It rapidly filled the road between steep banks. Snow fingers groped along the macadam, clutching the road and closing it as snow blew in from the fields.

I turned to Anna. "This is as far as we drive. Less than a mile to meet Martin."

"We can't walk through that mess." Anna grimaced. "They wouldn't find our bodies for a week."

"Only one possibility." I nodded toward the outline of a small house near the road. "A young Mennonite couple live here. We'll get William out of bed. His wife is due in March. He'll understand."

Gasping for breath against the wind, I floundered through a drift, removed a glove and pounded on an outer door with an intensity that rattled windows and vibrated the frame house.

"William! William! Wake up! I need help. William Burkholder wake up!" I shouted.

Finally, in a back room, I saw the faint glow of a match become the flame of a lamp. William shuffled from the sleeping room, pulling suspenders over his nightshirt. He walked into the kitchen and peered through the window with a bewildered look.

"Who's out there?" He raised his lamp to the glass.

"Me. Dr. Kaiser."

He unbolted the door and I stepped into the kitchen, taking a snow shower along.

"What are you doing out tonight?" William rubbed sleepy eyes and shook his tousled head.

"Can you hitch up and take Anna and me to meet Martin Weaver at the next crossroad?" I asked, watching William drag himself into consciousness. "It's baby night for them."

"Yes, of course." He smiled with comprehension. "But we've only been married a year. All we have is a buggy with one seat."

"Fine," I said, for I would have ridden a wheelbarrow.

"I'll get dressed and hitch up."

I could hear William speaking in low tones to his wife as he exchanged bare feet for boots and his muslin nightshirt for outdoor clothes.

My face burned with cold as I wallowed back to Anna. When we heard the harnessed horse clatter iron shoes on the stones at the barn forebay, we wrapped mufflers around our faces and moved into the storm.

"Too bad you have to be out tonight," William said. He pulled a thick coat collar against the ear flaps on his black leather hat, helped me onto the buggy seat, and set the bag behind my legs. Anna sat on my lap and William beside me. He threw a heavy lap robe over us. With only our eyes showing above heavy scarves, we looked like a trio of bandits.

"Up Sue. Giddy up," William shouted, slapping the reins over her back. She stood still. "Go Sue," he shouted louder.

She jumped forward, nearly throwing us backward over the seat. "Hope it doesn't get too deep. Sometimes horses lie down in deep drifts," William said anxiously as the buggy lights shone through blowing snow clouds.

There was no conversation except William urging his mare forward. I gripped Anna with one hand, the seat with the other. We pitched and heaved at precarious angles. It seemed that we would upset or Sue might flounder in the snow.

Anna was no lightweight. She became heavier as we bounced. I braced both feet against the floorboards until my legs became numb. Anna's body shielded my eyes from the cutting snow which nearly blinded her and William. It froze to their eyebrows and hung on their lashes.

Our driver gave full attention to his animal as she slowly struggled through the draw. When the snow came to Sue's belly, William leaned forward, slapped the reins on her back, and shouted, "Gid up Sue." She strained through drift after drift. The muscles of her hindquarters stretched taut beneath gray hide as she pulled into the harness.

It seemed hours, but the half mile could have lasted no more than 20 minutes before we reached the far ridge and the crossroad where Martin waited, a black speck in a white sea.

Transfer of passengers was brief. William, aware of Martha's labor, was shy and reserved. He seemed happy to turn Sue toward home and a warm bed.

"Hi, Kaiser. Good ta see ya. There's no hurry," Martin shouted above the wailing wind. "The missus thinks she'll have it tonight. Better ta get ya in plenty a time."

Martin slid open the side door of his carriage and set my bag inside. He held his wide-brimmed hat in a battle with the storm, which whipped his long black coat and blew its cape over his head.

"Get in back with your bag," Martin yelled. "It'll be rough riding tonight. Road's closed. We'll go through the fields." He spit a dark spurt into the snow and shifted the lump in his cheek.

I placed a boot on the carriage's iron step and slid onto the back bench behind a folded seat. Martin's words, "Thinks she'll have it tonight," beat in my ears.

"Let's hope this isn't a dry run," Anna said, unfolding the front seat.

Martin checked something on the harness, sat on a seat beside Anna, and closed both side doors. He picked up the dangling reins. "Get up Bud," he called from within his great coat.

The Weavers were an older established Mennonite family and owned a closed wagon. It was a welcome refuge. These market wagons seemed like large matchboxes set on four wheels and covered with black rubberized canvas. The reins entered through holes where two glass panels met the lower wooden dashboard. Beside each front seat a door with a glass panel slid inside the canvas back half. In summer, the canvas rear panel could be rolled up or removed.

Carriages were built for transportation, not comfort. Protection from jolts were two large inadequate leaf springs. It was the near lack of springs which impressed me the night of the blizzard.

Martin clucked to Bud, turned into Abner Huyard's field, and headed west.

Crop rotation is an important factor in Lancaster County's agricultural success. If only Abner had rotated

alfalfa, wheat, or potatoes in his large corner field the previous summer, or if he had planted his corn rows east to
west instead of north to south, I would not have thought
about wagon springs.

The frost was two feet deep. Bud, headed home, thought
nothing of the carriage behind him. Each cornrow was a
rocky mountain, separated by deep valleys into which we
fell with a thud over and over. A rhythmic jarring of teeth
and bones. The wagon shook and rattled as if falling apart.
I hoped the wheels had been hooped and tightened recently.

Except for the blizzard's heavy breath rising and falling
around us, the only noise was the wagon bouncing over the
corrugated field. I felt displaced into a Victorian novel.

Suddenly a giggle erupted from the red coat. Another
and another followed. Then uncontrolled hiccups. Anna
shook with laughter.

I, too, began to laugh.

Martin, apparently immune to humor and not in tune
with giggling women, braced himself against the floorboards. He hunched forward trying to see through the
frosted windshield. Occasionally he held the wiper handle
and moved its blade across the clouded glass.

Bud was allowed to hunt his way home. Suddenly he
jerked to a stop.

"What now?" Martin asked.

"There's a creek out there," I said peeking through the
patch of side window. "The horse has his chest against a
fence."

"Creek? There's no creek around here!" Martin shouted.
He flung a gloved hand across Anna and slid open the side
door with such unexpected force that I felt my nose had

been sheared from my face.

"Well, there's one out there tonight," I said, between laughter and pain. I patted the injured appendage with a gloved hand. No blood.

"I've never been down here before," Martin admitted.

"Never been north of the crossroad?" Anna hiccupped.

"We've wandered downhill to Abner's cow pasture," I told Martin. "I can make out his water wheel in the creek. We better go the other way."

Martin headed the sorrel uphill. Again we bumped over each row. I felt scrubbed on a washboard. Finally, we came to windswept macadam before the Weaver home.

Hoary elms surrounded the old farmhouse. The storm lashed branches against the clapboards as if begging to go inside. Wind moaned and fell through naked limbs.

Martin helped us from the carriage into a hip-high drift encircling the house. We struggled into the kitchen, dimly lit by a small lamp casting dull shadows down a long table. I raised the flame.

Anna and I shook our wet coats and hung them on hooks behind a tepid cookstove. We knocked snow from our boots into the zinc-lined sink and hung scarves over chairbacks.

"Hello, there! What a night to bring you out," Martha called through the open bedroom door. "Guess I'll have this baby sometime tonight."

"We certainly hope so after that trip," I answered, still peeling off clothing. "Babies have no respect for bad weather."

I walked stocking-footed through the kitchen and bedroom over cold linoleum. A portable heater meagerly heated the sleeping room and gave off kerosene odors.

Only Martha's mottled-gray hair and flaccid face against the white bolster showed above the quilts, piled from high headboard to the footboard.

Barely past 36, Martha had birthed seven children and had had four miscarriages. A pale kerosene lamp accented furrows around her sagging chin and sad brown eyes.

I felt a hopelessness about this birth, and I thought of my baby daughter who brought such great pleasure into our lives. I unpacked my bag and examined Martha.

"Sometime tonight," I agreed.

"I will be glad to have it over," Martha said quietly, turning her face toward the wall. "The children will be happy for a new baby." She sighed and pulled the pink sheet blanket and quilts around her neck with thin fingers.

"Sun rises at 7:30," I said. "We'll see if you're right."

"Make yourselves comfortable in the kitchen."

During the night I decided that comfort is a relative term. The only heat in the barn-like kitchen came from the ancient iron cookstove, banked for the night.

Anna and I pulled two rocking chairs from a colder parlor, opened the oven door, and stuck our wet feet inside, hunting its skimpy heat for our frigid toes.

"Are ya cold?" Martin asked, stomping in from the barn. He hung his snow-crusted coat behind the stove, balanced his hat on its cape. They looked like a collapsed scarecrow.

Martin removed four-buckle arctics and shook snow onto the floor. He was gaunt and rangy without the great coat, his sharp features lean and lined. When he relaxed, crows-feet around his narrow mouth and pale eyes became white lines on a weary face.

The farmer pulled a paper from his denim pants and walked across the kitchen to a corner desk. He opened the lid and stuffed the scrap into a pigeonhole, already crammed full.

I wondered if the papers were bills.

When Martin stooped to retrieve a pen that had rolled onto the floor, I noticed expansive pink scalp in his wispy brown hair. He rubbed a calloused hand over his long stubble, glanced at us uneasily, then looked toward the bedroom with a longing I interpreted as a desire to lie down and finish sleeping.

"Why don't you rest with Martha," I suggested.

"Make yourselves comfortable," Martin's smile showed brown irregular teeth. Several were missing. "I'll make it warmer in here." Raising the upper tread of two steps that protruded into the room from a stairway, he picked out three sticks, dropped them onto coal in the firebox, and opened the draft slightly. Martin removed his workshoes, lay on the quilts beside Martha, covered himself with a blanket, and soon snored loudly.

"Here we sit like birds in the wilderness," Anna sang. She shivered and pulled the red coat around her sweatered shoulders.

Behind us the wind beat vinyl strips fastened outside the house to reduce winter drafts. They undulated and snapped with each gust. I lay on a worn couch beneath north windows, but air blew around the plastic and through the window frames. It was cold. I envied women asleep beside their husbands in warm beds.

Anna found glasses in the wooden cupboard and filled them from a hand pump at the sink. We warmed our drinks from a teakettle on the stove.

"Let's get more wood," Anna said when the stove cooled. We covertly fed the fire all night with wood from under the steps, listened to the storm, and catnapped. Occasionally we left our chairs and walked around the kitchen or sat at the table until cold drove us back to the stove.

I refused to dwell on the possibility of a birth complication in our uncompromising situation. When I checked Martha at five o'clock, I knew our vigil had not been wasted. Her moans, softer than those of the storm, grew louder. They were never as frantic or uncontrolled as the blizzard.

"Ugh, ugh. It's soon here," Martha grunted after seven o'clock.

Martin rushed to turn up the bedroom heater. He brought another one from the washhouse and piled wood into the kitchen stove. The rooms became warmer.

We heard children moving overhead. Martin called up the stairwell in Pennsylvania Dutch, ordering them to stay in the bedrooms. His word was law; they asked no questions.

Martin hung a brighter pressure lantern over the footboard. He sat on a chair near the bed. "Lie still. Push hard. It's soon over," he comforted Martha.

Amniotic fluid, an ellipse of wet hair, Martha's deep breath, and then a writhing, snorting baby girl lay on the bed as dawn's first glimmer shone in the east through the kitchen windows.

"We could have used another boy around her," Martin said, half in jest.

"Girls are better than boys," I teased, bumping my head on the lantern again. "They work in the house *and* barn."

Martin grinned. "But girls don't haul manure, and I don't know any man who likes that job." He laughed. "Maybe we'll have a boy next time."

Martha frowned. "I'm glad it's over. I was worried about being snowed in," she said to Anna who dressed the baby in warm clothes.

Ten years seemed to have dropped from Martha as if by magic. She glowed in the triumph of new birth, moved sprightly in the bed as I helped her into a fresh flannel nightgown warmed at the stove. "I can't wait for the children to see their new sister. The last baby is three already."

"Don't you mind the extra work?" I asked.

"No. I have plenty of my own help this time, and there's no outside work now." She hugged the new baby.

Martin lifted the green window shades, pulled to sills against cold wind. Morning sun dazzled the snow with glaring brilliance. Across the landscape, shadowed drifts rose and fell. Fence rows lifted the shimmering white like pulsing blood vessels.

The storm was finished. Windless trees stood mute beside the house. Unmarred snow mantled the countryside.

Time to go home.

Alta, 16, came to care for her mother and prepare the family breakfast.

Martin again hitched Bud to the market wagon. He hustled us out of the house before the other children came downstairs.

This time we drove across the Weaver's hay field to Shirk Road. We followed tracks along its banks where other travelers had already cut fences. Ahead, bells jingled on horses pulling a bobsled. In the draw where William had driven the night before, snow filled the 12-foot banks.

Houses and barns freckled the sun-drizzled hills. I wondered how many days would pass before plows cleared the blizzard from back roads, how many tons of milk dairymen would pour onto the ground before trucks could pick up their loads again. Picture-postcard serenity embraced the land.

Serenity also embraced my station wagon. All night the driving snow had sifted under its hood. The engine refused to start. William wallowed through drifts to bring a neighbor with his tractor and heavy chain. He towed us to New Holland Pike, now one lane through heavy drifts. Finally the engine turned over and we sputtered home.

By mid-morning, I sat in my warm kitchen. I wearily removed my boots. Pete walked past humming a cheerful tune. He carried a shovel and guided two boisterous children padded in snowsuits.

"Have a good night, dear?" he asked.

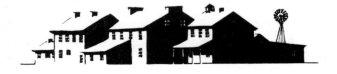

19.
Identity

Mary Petersheim, wife of Isaac B., or was it Mattie Petersheim—John Z., lunched under the ancient apple tree in our backyard. She rose and brushed crumbs and September leaves clinging to her black dress and stockings. I watched her barefooted preschoolers gather bag and wrappings before the four tramped across the browning lawn toward the front street and waiting room.

I set my lunch plate in the sink and wondered if Mattie, or was it Mary, had lunched on balogna, too. Had she been as generous with the mustard?

There was good reason to confuse Amish names and people. Thousands lived in a community centering in Lancaster County. Approximately 16 family names and a limited number of given names were repeated over and over. Every family seemed to have a John, Sam, Mary, and Susie. The Amish themselves had identification problems and referred frequently to *The Fisher Book* of genealogy to sort out kinships.

Old Order Mennonite families with the many Goods, Martins, Burkholders, Zimmermans, Nolts, and Weavers were as confusing. I smiled, thinking rural mail carriers should lobby for a "Limitation of Names Bill."

The day was a sunny Monday after three days of steady rain. Fields were too wet for work, and the weekly horse sale encouraged men to bring their families into town for shopping and doctor visits. My driveway was rimmed with cars of many vintages and colors, mostly black. An assortment of stomping horses with buggies, wagons, and carts was tied to the hitching rail.

The white paneled door dividing husband, children, and cooking from the world of patients, pills, and bandages closed behind me.

"Anyone in labor today?" nurse Anna asked. "I can't find a chart for Mary S. Stoltzfus—John S. from Smoketown. Looked through all 20 Mary Stoltzfuses up here. I'll look in the old files in the basement. Sure hope you don't get called out of the office today. When they can't plow they come to the doctor like fleas to a hound."

Mary Petersheim passed in from the waiting room to the toilet with two of her children. When the door opened it looked as though all the afternoon appointments had arrived early. Every chair was taken. Squirmy babies slithered on mothers' laps, sucked cloudy bottles, or bobbled pacifiers. Several children sat on the floor ripping pages from magazines. In the corner chair Malinda Zook folded her sandwich wrapper to use on another trip to town. The Abbott pharmaceutical salesman shrank into his chair amid the Pennsylvania Dutch words flying between women darning socks, nursing babies, and embroidering. The room hummed like bees in a June clover field.

"Yes," I said, "Susie Beiler, John S., is in labor. Just checked her an hour ago. Probably won't need me until tonight. Look at that mess out there. I wonder how many Extras today?" I looked through a small one-way mirrored window.

Extras came in three categories. One kind merely occupied a chair. They tagged along with a patient because they either had errands in town or nothing better to do.

The second Extra came with a patient who had an appointment. They were certain the doctor would be delighted to also care for their interesting and urgent medical problem. Today these would get little or none of my time.

Extra Number Three really needed a physician's care, hadn't taken time to telephone for an appointment, but knew their condition needed immediate attention. This kind were disastrous on a busy day. Patients knew I was too soft to turn them away.

As I walked into the front examining room I heard small children running across the wooden porch and saw, through the slanted Venetian blinds, several men sitting on the porch wall. They probably talked of uncut hay or prognosticated this year's tobacco prices. Several blew decisive smoke clouds from chimney-fat cigars or spat emphatically into the juniper bushes.

By 1:30 I had seen Malinda Zook's rounded abdomen, given the Reiff baby its three-month checkup, treated Henry Martin's lumbago, and was removing stitches from Martha Zimmerman's hand when Anna interrupted us.

"John S. Beiler just called. He said you're to come right away. Hurry. He doesn't know if you can make it in time. He hung up so he could run home."

Within moments I finished the hand and left the office. The waiting room party broke up, either to reconvene after shopping trips in town or on another day.

The straightest roads in Lancaster County point like spokes of a wheel toward Lancaster City, the hub. From New Holland these were east and west highways. Today I drove south over meandering cow paths that wound around fields, churches, and tobacco patches, along wandering meadow streams and over hilltops like thread from a runaway spool.

In my stork race there was no time to think of the autumn sunshine falling on stubbled fields of shocked corn, standing sentinel to pungent patches of newly mown hay. No time to notice the rows of last tobacco that stretched broad green arms toward the sun. Fallow brown acres waited drills of winter wheat. Each sloped plot bordered against the next, separated only by farm lane or wire fence until they ended at short-cropped cow pastures with spindly brooks. From these streams another ramp of fields climbed hills fringed with trees hinting of fall colors.

The rolling countryside repeated this mold over and over as if stamped by some great mystical machine. Scattered farms and villages interrupted the pattern and delighted the eye.

From the town of Intercourse I sped eastward on the Old Philadelphia Pike through the hamlets of Spring Garden, White Horse, and Cains. I straddled rutted furrows cut into the macadam by sharp-shod horses, dodged unconcerned pedestrians and slow horses pulling ragged loads of corn on the way to buzzing silo fillers. I zipped past slow-driving old men in antiquated cars taxiing Amish on errands.

At Cains I headed north at the old hotel, bouncing in

potholes and snaking around barns. I kept repeating my motto—"Either late or sit and wait." Cleaning up when I arrived late could be worse than waiting.

Dust flew into asters and petunias when I came to a quick stop at the Beiler yard fence. Black bag in hand, I ran up a long concrete walk and into Beilers' big farm kitchen. Everything was neat and orderly. The sink and drainboard were clean. Dish towels hung on their rack. No Susie.

In a quick vision I saw the patient lying in bed, baby wrapped in towels on her abdomen, John hovering, proud of his obstetrical job and claiming the fee.

Snapping jar lids boomed like cannon in the hollow house. I rushed over spotless linoleum to the bedroom doorway beyond the gas stove. Susie's high-headed oak bed was as vacant and clean-sheeted as when I had seen it several hours before. On the dresser stood a new bottle of baby lotion, a gray enamel wash basin, my printed instructions, and a neat pile of baby clothes. Everything was ominously quiet.

A new vision. Now I knew. Another bathroom baby. Maybe Susie alone, in trouble.

"Susie!" I called anxiously. "Where are you?"

I pictured her lying on the concrete floor, head on a needlepoint chair cushion, blanketed baby on her belly.

"Susie!" I called again, running through the kitchen into the kettlehouse where a bathroom had been built into one corner several years ago when the drafty two-holer was abandoned.

"Hello! What are you doing her?" Startle-eyed, Susie stood in the bathroom. She paused in mid-step. Alone in the house and in labor, she wore no cape or apron over a brown dress that clung to her distended abdomen like freshly poured molasses and exaggerated her stubby roundness. Brown hair, pulled into a coil at the back of her head, was covered with a tightly drawn blue bandana handkerchief. Her thin lips twisted to a puzzled grin. "What are you doing here?" she repeated.

"John called, said I was to come in a hurry."

"Not my John. He's out raking hay. I sent the kids to brother Stevie's. If I need John I'm to hang a sheet on the clothesline. Nothing's changed. Probably tonight sometime."

Susie swayed across the kettlehouse, slapping bare feet on the smooth concrete floor. They kept time with my pounding heart. I could see her sly smile and the laughter in her eyes. What fun. A joke on the doctor. Went to the wrong house.

"Thought you had office hours now," she said, pretending to inspect the cooling tomatoes while she savored my discomfort.

"Where is there another John S. Beiler?" I asked, stunned, panicked, embarrassed. I leaned languidly against the doorjamb, but my bag would not remain still in nervous hands. Mouth dry, my voice rose to a pleading whine. "Is there another John S. Beiler?"

Susie walked to the sink, rinsed her hands, scratched her bleb of a nose, carefully dried her fingers on a towel behind the kettlehouse door, and finally answered. "I believe you must want John S. and Malinda Beiler near Hess' Mill. Hope you make it."

Now she was privy to a guarded secret, the identity of a laboring woman. Numerous times I was asked to park behind a shadowy barn or corncrib so passing neighbors did not recognize my station wagon.

"Thank you. See you later, Susie," I called, running down the mile-long walk. White and purple aster petals fluttered to the ground when the yard gate slammed against its fence. Ripe blue grapes smashed onto the concrete from an overhead arbor. Everything seemed to laugh.

Bouncing in six directions like a dried pea in a pod, I sped back to Cains. The Old Philadelphia Pike seemed no smoother at illegal speeds. Near the Cattails I turned south onto a twisting narrow road past Hershey Mennonite Church to the Newport Road near Hess' Feed Mill.

Which would it be, I wondered, stopping abruptly at the base of a high earthen bank—wait or clean-up? My hand gripped the black bag as tightly as it had the steering wheel. Bounding up 15 wooden steps that seemed like 115, I stopped to catch my breath on a broad porch. John, a bulky farmer in patched and faded broadfalls, relaxed lazily against the wide stone doorway, one thumb tucked under a suspender. His cuffless pants had shrunk well above bare feet and bony ankles. One big toe wore a once-white generous bandage tied in a thick knot on top the foot.

He uncrossed his legs and stepped forward, opening the sagging wooden screen door with a brown muscular arm. A dangling tail of cotton, tied to the screen to scare away flies, flapped at the motion. It was kinked from confinement in a bottle.

John's thin face appeared as somber as a thunderstorm about to break. He was silent, irritated. He towered above me like a stone monument. At least six foot four, I thought. Suddenly his mouth twitched. His blue eyes shone and he exploded a hearty, happy laugh. "No need to hurry. Where you been, Doc? I get the fee this time."

"Got here soon as possible," I said limply. Amish gossip would report the truth soon enough. I followed John through a work-littered kitchen, a hurricane disaster area. Kettles with and without lids sat on the black gas stove, some steaming the pungent odor of hot grapes. A disarray of empty canning jars filled the sink. Buckets of grapes stood beside the long table. Lids, spoons, and diapers lay everywhere and anywhere. Sugar in a hundred-pound bag sat beside the stove.

"Hi, Doc. What took you so long?" Malinda asked, squinting through narrowed lids, as she did when excited. She smiled, relaxing her eyes into azure marbles. A blanketed baby, loudly sucking its fist, snuffled on her abdomen. Malinda lay in the expected murky puddle fully dressed.

"Work's all done. I get paid this time." John's tanned face sparked the triumphant smile seen more times than made me comfortable.

"Guess you don't need me then." I picked up my bag as if to leave. "Looks like John has everything under control."

"Well, as long as you're here," John laughed, feigning helplessness.

"I was too busy in the grapes to call sooner. I always go fast. I just wasn't expecting this baby today with all those grapes to do up," Malinda said, patting the baby.

"Maybe we can split the fee." John, in field-smudged clothes, hovered and goaded while I delivered the placenta and handed it to him for burial in the garden away from animals or curious children.

Their son was soon weighed, cleaned, and dressed. "Watch carefully and you can do it all next time," I said. "Will you please go to the mill and call my office. Tell them

I'll return in an hour."

"Might as well do it all. I did the important part," he laughed, leaving through the back door.

"I was in labor less than an hour. You couldn't possibly have gotten here in time," Malinda confided as I helped slide her petite body out of the wet dress and into the shower beside the bedroom.

"You'll soon feel fine," I said stretching clean sheets across the bed.

"Look at me." She held up hands purple from fingertip to arm. Grape splotches freckled her childlike face and slender arms. Both feet were mottled purple from helping the children pick grapes beneath the arbor.

Malinda soon rested in a dry bed. She could not force loose strands of dark hair under her cap. They escaped everywhere from the once-tight center part and coiled knot. Exasperated, she tugged at the thick chestnut rope until it fell loosely over her shoulder and across the pillow. She reached for her baby and suckled him at her breast.

John returned from the mill and sat on a chair beside Malinda. He also sat on my instructions: "What to Do If the Baby Beats the Doctor." With a large calloused hand, he gently touched his wife's shoulder, caressed the baby along its head, lifted a tiny fist until it gripped his big finger.

Timidly, Malinda stretched a lavender hand across her chest and rested it softly on John's a moment. "Another fine healthy boy. We can be thankful."

"Malinda, your maiden name was Stoltzfus," I said, recording information for the birth certificate. "That will probably give the baby 'S.' for a middle initial. Do you and John have a first name yet?"

She raised onto an elbow toward John with a resolved

and triumphant smile. Her eyes narrowed, face tensed. "After six boys maybe we'll have a girl next time if we call this one Junior. John deserves a namesake when he delivers the baby. We'll call him John—John S. Beiler."

A Word About These People . . .

The Mennonites and Amish are much like an extended family. With many branches, each with its own particularities, the groups are still more alike than different.

The Amish and Mennonites have common faith rooting. Their beginning can be traced to the Protestant Reformation in 16th-century Europe. In 1525, a group of believers parted company with the established state church for a variety of reasons. Among them was the conviction that one must voluntarily become a follower of Christ, and that that deliberate decision will be reflected in all of one's life. Therefore, baptism must symbolize that choice. The movement was nicknamed "Anabaptism," meaning re-baptism, since the believers wanted to be baptized again as adults.

Eventually these people were called Mennonites after Menno Simons, one of their leaders who had formerly been a Roman Catholic priest. Over the years they grew into a strong faith community, concerned with the nurture and discipline of each other.

Basic to their beliefs was a conviction that if one was a faithful follower of Christ's, one's behavior would clearly distinguish one from the larger world. These people saw themselves as "separated unto God" because of their values of love, forgiveness, and peace. Because they were misunderstood and because they appeared to be a threat to the established church and government, the people were often persecuted and many became refugees.

In 1693, a charismatic young Mennonite leader, Jacob Amman, believed that the church was losing some of its purity and that it was beginning to compromise with the world. And so he and a group who agreed with him left the Mennonites and formed a separate fellowship. They were called Amish, after their leader. Today the Amish identify themselves as the most conservative group of Mennonites.

Both the Mennonites and Amish have split and realigned many times throughout the years. In some cases, personality conflicts were the reasons. But most often the concerns were about the need for maintaining purity and faithfulness within the church. How that should be done and to what degree are the critical questions that have often resulted in division.

While the various Mennonite and Amish groups have few doctrinal differences, they differ most in specific practices. In general, the Amish tend to be more wary of interchange with the larger world. They are more distinctly separate in lifestyle. The Old Order Amish do not own or drive cars, they live without electricity, have prescribed dress patterns, operate their own schools, and speak Pennsylvania Dutch among themselves, a language which further defines their group. They are also cautious about doing missions.

In general, the Mennonites have been more open to give-and-take with the larger world, accepting technology and education, being less distinctively different in lifestyle, and being active in mission work. They have fostered group identity by working at making church central to

social life, and allowing their Christian faith to be the moti-
vation for one's training or choice of job, or how one uses
money.

But none of these are static people. Nor are these gener-
alizations categorically true. There are Amish groups who
use technology and promote higher learning. And there are
Mennonites who drive horses and buggies, follow noncon-
formity in their dress, and prefer farm-related occupations.

For instance, the Amish Mennonite groups, sometimes
called the Beachy Amish after their founder, have vigorous
mission programs. And although their dress patterns
reflect their Old Order Amish connections, they drive cars,
use electricity, and many send their children to high
school.

The Old Order Mennonite group, nicknamed Wenger
Mennonites after their leader, drive horses and carriages,
dress very distinctively and do not actively practice missions. Another Old Order Mennonite group, the Horning
Mennonites, do drive cars, but with the chrome painted
black in many cases, and have electricity in their homes.

The total North American membership of all groups in
this Anabaptist "family of faith" now surpasses 400,000.
About 62,000 of these are Old Order Amish, scattered in
clusters throughout 21 states and one Canadian province.
The second largest of these communities is found in
Lancaster County in eastern Pennsylvania, the setting of
Dr. Frau. Members of Amish, Mennonite, and other
Anabaptist groups comprise about one-tenth of Lancaster
County's total population.

About the Author

Grace H. Kaiser practiced medicine in New Holland, a town in eastern Lancaster County, Pennsylvania, for 28 years. During that time she was also on the staffs of the Lancaster Osteopathic and Ephrata Community hospitals.

A native of Bucks County, Pennsylvania, she is a graduate of the College of Chestnut Hill and The Philadelphia College of Osteopathic Medicine.

Dr. Kaiser became disabled in October, 1978, and had to retire from practice. (She chronicles that experience in the book, *Detour.*) Today, she is retired in Phoenix, Arizona. She and her late husband Peter are the parents of four grown children and the grandparents of three.